First and Second Series

MULTIPLE CHOICE TUTOR

Basic Sciences in OBSTETRICS and GYNAECOLOGY

V. R. TINDALL MD, MSc, FRCS, FRCOG

Professor of Obstetrics and Gynaecology, University of Manchester

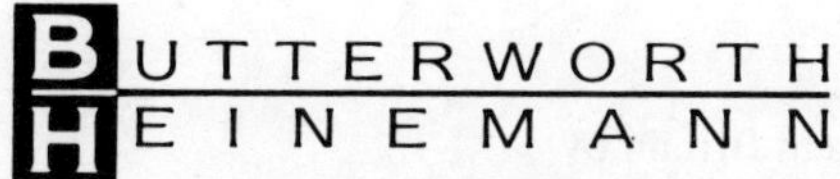

Butterworth-Heinemann Ltd
Linacre House, Jordan Hill, Oxford OX2 8DP

PART OF REED INTERNATIONAL BOOKS

OXFORD LONDON BOSTON
MUNICH NEW DELHI SINGAPORE SYDNEY
TOKYO TORONTO WELLINGTON

Formerly published in two volumes:
MCQ Tutor: MRCOG Part 1 Basic Sciences as Applied to Obstetrics and Gynaecology 1977, 1980
MCQ Tutor: Basic Sciences in Obstetrics and Gynaecology Second Series 1985

First published 1987
Reprinted 1988, 1990, 1992

British Library Cataloguing in Publication Data
Tindall, V. R.
Basic sciences in obstetrics and gynaecology
(Multiple choice tutor. First and second series)
1. Gynaecology – examinations, questions, etc.
2. Obstetrics – examinations, questions, etc.
I. Title II. Series
610'.246181 RG111

ISBN 0 7506 0784 X

Printed and bound in Great Britain by
Biddles Ltd, Guildford and King's Lynn

FIRST SERIES

CONTENTS

FOREWORD

Examinations involving multiple choice questions have become familiar to us all in recent years. Familiarity, however, does not in this respect breed contempt. To candidates all examinations, whatever their form, are a matter for anxiety, which is partly due to uncertainty in the candidate's mind about what the examiners are looking for. This book explains simply and clearly what is involved in MCQ examinations; it shows how questions are devised and what marking system is employed. It provides an opportunity for the candidate to familiarise himself with the type of question asked and the fields covered as well as to test himself to determine his own progress. The book is directed principally to the Part 1 examination for membership of the Royal College of Obstetricians and Gynaecologists, but it is applicable, too, to other similar examinations.

I am delighted that such an excellent book has been produced by Professor Tindall on behalf of the Royal College of Obstetricians and Gynaecologists. I feel it will be a great success.

Professor Sir John Dewhurst,
immediate past President: Royal College of Obstetricians & Gynaecologists
August 1977

INTRODUCTION

The purpose of this Tutor Book, as other books in this series, is primarily an aid to teaching and learning. Whilst it is aimed at helping potential Obstetricians and Gynaecologists, some of the sections will benefit other postgraduates. An attempt has been made to present questions which are based on a broad knowledge of the basic sciences, as applied in their widest sense to medical practice. The aspects covered in certain subjects, e.g. anatomy, have been deliberately restricted to the area, or systems, of the body considered appropriate for training the modern Obstetrician and Gynaecologist.

In essence, the subjects covered will be those required for the Part 1 MRCOG, and equivalent examinations, namely; anatomy, biochemistry, cell biology, embryology, endocrinology, elementary statistics, genetics, immunology, microbiology, pathology, pharmacology and physiology. In multiple choice questions (MCQ's) there is often an overlap of subject material within an individual question. The decision as to which section a question has been allocated is purely that of the Author. Some of the topics mentioned above have been grouped together for convenience, and the sections contain a variable number of questions. It does not reflect the pattern of any examination, merely the ease with which suitable questions could be devised.

It is well known to those actually involved in their preparation that, in order to obtain good MCQ's it takes a lot of time and hard work. It usually involves a small number of individuals who have acquired the ability, after considerable effort, and the questions presented are no exception. Most of the MCQ's have been considered by a small group of Fellows, or Members, of the Royal College of Obstetricians and Gynaecologists, or co-opted experts in a particular field of basic sciences initially. After considerable alteration of the original questions, they appear in a modified form in an examination. The subsequent analysis and review of their performance has resulted, in many instances, in further alterations in order to avoid ambiguity or improve the question. In some instances, the material has had to be updated in light of further knowledge, or changes in units of measurement, i.e. SI units. It is hoped that by providing answers and comments, this book will provide a useful aid to learning, or relearning, the techniques of answering multiple choice questions. It must be emphasised that no book of MCQ's, even with answers, should be taken in isolation, it must be used in conjunction with the appropriate text books.

Answer sheets are included at the back of the book, so that the reader can complete them before looking at the answers, if so wished. The five part answer format used in this book is that used for many higher examinations in the United Kingdom. Each question starts with an initial statement or word ('stem'), followed by five possible completions or ('items'). It is planned that all the answers are equally possible and do not include any mutually exclusive items. The reader has to decide, wherever possible, which item is true and which is false. For marking purposes, the reader should allocate one mark (+1) for the appropriate correct answer. One mark should be deducted (−1) for each incorrect answer. No mark (0) is given for not answering or attempting an individual item. In each of the questions, any number of items may be correct, although in this book it is only very occasionally that all five items are either correct or incorrect. Since some questions contain factual items of knowledge, which any reasonable candidate for the Part 1 MRCOG should get correct, the aim for the potential candidate should be about 60% of the marks for the number of questions chosen by the reader.

Despite the continual criticism of examinations, they are still a necessary hurdle in a medical career, and MCQ papers are merely one of the methods of assessment of ability. There will always be reservations about the merits of MCQ's by the examiners and candidates involved. It is therefore hoped that whilst this book will primarily help potential candidates to obtain some knowledge and practice in the format currently used, it may also be of some help to those Consultants and Specialists who are responsible for their training.

1. ANATOMY

1.1. In the femoral triangle, the femoral artery:

- **A.** Lies anterior to the genital branch of the genito-femoral nerve
- **B.** Lies medial to the femoral nerve
- **C.** Is separated by the femoral vein from the psoas muscle
- **D.** Is crossed anteriorly by the superficial circumflex iliac vein
- **E.** Lies medial to the femoral vein

1.2. In the normal human pelvis:

- **A.** The promontory of the sacrum is the upper anterior border of the first sacral vertebra
- **B.** The sacrum has four paired foramina anteriorly
- **C.** The obturator foramen is covered completely by a membrane
- **D.** The pubic bone contributes to the formation of the acetabular fossa
- **E.** The ischial spines are situated anterior to the respective obturator foramen

1.3. In the os innomminatum (hip bone):

- **A.** Its three constituent bones meet in the acetabulum
- **B.** The greater sciatic notch forms a more acute angle in the female
- **C.** The acetabulum is smaller in the female
- **D.** The ischial spine is situated on the anterior border of the ischium
- **E.** The joint between the pubic bones is synovial in type

Answers overleaf

1.1. B, D.

The femoral artery lies posterior to the genital branch of the genito-femoral nerve. The femoral vein is a medial relation of the artery and the artery lies on the psoas muscle.

1.2. A, B, D.

The obturator membrane nearly closes the obturator foramen, it does not completely cover the foramen. Each ischial spine is situated posterior to the respective obturator foramen.

1.3. A, C.

One of the characteristic sex differences is that the greater sacrosciatic notch is more acute in the male. The ischial spine is situated on the posterior border of the ischium. The joint between the pubic bones is a cartilaginous joint although it does have a disc of fibrocartilage between the two bones. The characteristic features of a synovial joint are given in question **1.11**.

1.4. The sacrotuberous ligament:

A. Is attached by its apex to the spine of the ischium
B. Is attached by its base to the posterior iliac spines
C. Gives origin to fibres of the gluteus maximus on its posterior surface
D. Forms the lower boundary of the greater sciatic foramen
E. Is continued along the ischial tuberosity as the falciform process

1.5. The following structures leave the pelvis by passing through the greater sciatic foramen above the piriformis muscle:

A. The sciatic nerve
B. The superior gluteal nerve
C. The internal pudendal vessels
D. The nerve to quadratus femoris muscle
E. The nerve to obturator internus

1.6. The ischio-rectal fossa:

A. Is directly related to the rectum on the medial side
B. Contains the perineal nerve in its posterior part
C. Is limited posteriorly by the gluteus maximus muscle
D. Communicates with the contralateral fossa posterior to the anus
E. Is separated from the ischium by the obturator externus muscle

Answers overleaf

1.4. B, C, E.

The sacrotuberous ligament is attached to the medial margin of the ischial tuberosity. It forms the medial boundary of the greater sciatic foramen and the lower boundary of the lesser sciatic foramen.

1.5. B.

All the structures mentioned pass below the piriformis muscle except the superior gluteal nerve (and vessels) which pass above the muscle.

1.6. B, C, D.

The medial wall of the ischio-rectal fossa consists of the pelvic diaphragm, the central tendon, and canal and ano-coccygeal ligament. The lateral wall is formed by the obturator internus, the ischial tuberosity and the sacro-tuberous ligament.

1.7. The levator ani muscle:

A. Is attached to the brim of the pelvis
B. Can act as a sphincter of the vagina
C. Has no attachment to the perineal body
D. Forms the roof of the ischio-rectal fossa
E. Has motor innervation from the pelvic autonomic nerves

1.8. The following muscles contribute to the perineal body:

A. External anal sphincter
B. Superficial transverse perineal muscle
C. Ischio-cavernosus
D. Pubococcygeus
E. Puborectalis

1.9. The iliac bone in the human female:

A. Gives origin of the psoas minor
B. Has two primary centres of ossification
C. Has two separate origins for the rectus femoris
D. Gives attachment to the sartorius muscle
E. Gives attachment to the inguinal ligament

Answers overleaf

1.7. B, D.

The levator ani is attached to the side wall of the true pelvis. The anterior fibres of the two levator ani muscles are attached to the perineal body. The muscle is supplied either by a branch of the fourth sacral nerve which arises from the inferior rectal nerve or from the perineal division of the pudendal nerve.

1.8. A, B, D.

Eight muscles converge and are attached to the anatomical perineal body: the external anal sphincter, the bulbospongiosus, the two superficial and deep transverse perineal muscles and the anterior fibres of the two levator ani.

1.9. C, D, E.

The psoas minor muscle is absent in about 40% of subjects. The psoas major would have been a better negative answer but since a question is included (**1.10**) on it the psoas minor was put in to remind the reader about it. When present it arises from the sides of the bodies of the twelfth thoracic and first lumbar vertebrae and from the disc in between them. It ends in a long, flat tendon which is inserted into the pecten pubis and iliopectinal eminence and by its lateral border into the iliac fascia. There is only one primary centre of ossification for the iliac bone.

1.10. The psoas major muscle:

A. Arises from the posterior surfaces of the transverse processes of the lumbar vertebrae
B. Is inserted into the lesser trochanter
C. Is covered anteriorly on the right side by the abdominal aorta
D. Acting from above flexes the thigh upon the pelvis
E. Acts as a lateral rotator of the femur

1.11. Characteristic features of a synovial joint are that:

A. The cartilage is eventually replaced by bone
B. It is completely surrounded by an articular capsule
C. Movement is impossible
D. The synovial membrane lines the whole of the interior of the joint
E. The joint cavity may be divided completely or incompletely by a fibrocartilaginous disc

1.12. The sheath of the rectus abdominis:

A. Is deficient posteriorly above the costal margin
B. Terminates below in the arcuate line
C. Is formed above the costal margin by the aponeurosis of the external oblique muscle
D. Forms the anterior wall of the inguinal canal
E. Separates the two rectus muscles at the linea semilunaris

Answers overleaf

1.10. B, D.

The psoas major arises from the anterior surfaces and lower borders of the transverse processes of all five lumbar vertebrae. The psoas major on the right side is covered by the inferior vena cava. The muscle does not act either as a medial or lateral rotator of the hip joint.

1.11. B, E.

The articular cartilage is not replaced by bone. Movement is always possible although the amount is variable. Most joints of the body including all the joints of the limb (except the tibiofibular syndesmosis and pubic symphysis) belong to the synovial group. The synovial membrane lines most of the interior of the joint cavity – the exception is the cartilage covered ends of the articulating bones.

1.12. A, C.

The sheath continues below the arcuate line since the aponeurosis of all three muscles pass in front of the rectus. The anterior wall of the inguinal canal has three distinct parts. It is formed laterally by both the muscular fibres of the internal oblique and the aponeurosis of the external oblique, its central part consists of the external oblique alone and medially it is deficient, at the superficial inguinal ring. The medial border of the rectus muscle is closely related to the linea alba. The lateral border is marked on the surface of the anterior abdominal wall by a curved groove termed the linea semilunaris which extends from the tip of the ninth costal cartilage to the pubic tubercle.

1.13. The vagina:

- **A.** Is partly developed from the urogenital sinus
- **B.** The external part of the muscular coat has longitudinal fibres
- **C.** Is lined by squamous epithelium
- **D.** Is covered posteriorly by pelvic peritoneum in its upper and middle thirds
- **E.** Derives its blood supply from the internal pudendal and vaginal arteries only

1.14. In the normal cervix:

- **A.** The canal is lined by transitional epithelium
- **B.** The level of the squamo-columnar junction varies at different periods of life
- **C.** The stroma is more fibrous than the body of the uterus
- **D.** Small cysts of the ectocervix are normal and common
- **E.** Keratinised stratified squamous epithelium is found over the vaginal aspect of the cervix

1.15. In veins:

- **A.** There are sympathetic nerves
- **B.** The blood flow fluctuates with the pulse
- **C.** Blood flow in the venae cava is increased during expiration
- **D.** There is elastic tissue
- **E.** There is the same endothelium as in arteries

Answers overleaf

1.13. A, B, C.

Posteriorly the peritoneum covers only the upper third of the vagina. It reccives arterial blood from the vaginal, uterine, internal pudendal and middle rectal branches of the internal iliac artery.

1.14. B, C, D.

The cervical canal is lined by a mucous membrane which consists of ciliated columnar epithelium in the upper two thirds of the canal. Transitional epithelium occurs in the ureters and the bladder. The normal epithelium of the cervix is not keratinised.

1.15. A, B, D.

Blood flow in the venae cava is increased in inspiration allowing an increased return of blood to the heart. Whilst there are similarities in the endothelium in veins and arteries there are also characteristic differences and therefore not identical.

1.16. The great (long) saphenous vein:

A. Contains no valves
B. Arises in the lateral marginal vein of the foot
C. Passes between the two heads of the gastrocnemius muscle
D. Is joined by the superficial epigastric vein
E. Lies behind the saphenous nerve in the leg

1.17. Branches of the femoral artery include the:

A. Superficial circumflex iliac artery
B. Deep external pudendal artery
C. Deep circumflex iliac artery
D. Inferior epigastric artery
E. Profunda femoris artery

Answers overleaf

1.16. D, E.

It is the longest vein in the body and begins in the medial margin vein of the foot. It contains about 10 – 20 valves which are more numerous in the leg than the thigh. In practically its entire extent the vein lies in the superficial fascia, but it has many communications with the deep veins especially in the leg.

1.17. A, B, E.

The deep circumflex iliac artery arises from the lateral side of the external iliac artery nearly opposite the inferior epigastric artery. The inferior epigastric artery arises from the external iliac artery immediately above the inguinal ligament.

1.18. Branches of the internal iliac artery include the:

A. Iliolumbar artery
B. Inferior vesical artery
C. Superior rectal artery
D. Middle rectal artery
E. Lateral sacral artery

1.19. Branches of the superior mesenteric artery include the:

A. Right gastro-epiploic artery
B. Ileo-colic artery
C. Right colic artery
D. Left colic artery
E. Right ovarian artery

1.20. Direct branches of the coeliac trunk (axis) include the:

A. Splenic artery
B. Left gastro-epiploic artery
C. Gastroduodenal artery
D. Hepatic artery
E. Short gastric arteries

Answers overleaf

1.18. A, B, D, E.

The superior rectal artery is a continuation of the inferior mesenteric artery.

1.19. B, C.

The right gastro-epiploic artery is the larger terminal branch of the gastro-duodenal artery. The left colic artery is a branch of the inferior mesenteric artery. Both ovarian arteries are direct branches of the abdominal aorta.

1.20. A, D.

The coeliac trunk has 3 branches, the left gastric, the hepatic and splenic arteries. The left gastro-epiploic artery is the largest branch of the splenic artery. The gastro-duodenal artery is a branch of the hepatic artery. The short gastric arteries are from 5 – 7 small branches which arise either from the end of the splenic artery and its terminal divisions or from the left gastro-epiploic artery.

1.21. The ureter in the adult human female:

A. Is lined in its upper two-thirds by transitional epithelium and in its lower one-third by columnar epithelium
B. On the left side enters the pelvis by crossing the left common iliac artery 2–3 cm above its bifurcation
C. The right ureter is usually more closely related to the vaginal vault than the left
D. Is separated by the external iliac vein from the psoas muscle
E. The ureteric orifices inside the bladder are 1.5 cm apart

1.22. The ureter:

A. Lies postero-superior to the internal iliac artery on the side wall of the pelvis
B. Lies superior to the uterine artery as it passes through the base of the broad ligament
C. Is narrowest where it pierces the bladder wall
D. On the side wall of the pelvis lies medial to the obturator nerve and vessels
E. At the pelvic brim lies anterior to the ovarian vessels

1.23. The sacral plexus:

A. Receives no contribution from the fourth lumbar nerve
B. Lies posterior to the piriformis muscle
C. Lies anterior to the ureter on the right side
D. The nerve to the obturator internus arises from the anterior branches of the anterior rami of the fifth lumbar, the first and second sacral nerves
E. Includes the anterior division of the third sacral nerve

Answers overleaf

1.21. D.

The whole of the ureter is lined by transitional epithelium. The ureter enters the pelvis by crossing in front of either the end of the common or the beginning of the external iliac vessels. It is the left ureter which is usually more clearly related to the vaginal vault than the right. The ureteric orifices are about 5.0 cm apart in the distended bladder and about 2.5 cm in the empty bladder.

1.22. C, D.

The ureter lies in front of the internal iliac artery and the commencement of its anterior trunk. The ureter is inferior to the uterine artery. The ureter lies posterior to the ovarian vessels at the pelvic brim.

1.23. D, E.

The sacral plexus is formed by the lumbosacral trunk which comprises part of the anterior ramus of the fourth lumbar nerve and the whole of the anterior ramus of the fifth lumbar nerve as well as the anterior rami of the first, second and third sacral nerves. The plexus lies in front of the piriformis muscle and behind the ureter.

1.24. The first sacral nerve root contributes to the following:

A. The nerve to obturator internus
B. The nerves to levatores ani
C. The obturator nerve
D. The anterior tibial nerve
E. The pudendal nerve

1.25. The pelvic splanchnic nerves:

A. Contain parasympathetic visceral motor nerve fibres
B. Arise from the posterior primary rami of S2 and S3
C. Supply motor fibres to the descending colon
D. Inhibit the detrusor muscle of the bladder
E. Supply vasodilator fibres to the erectile tissue of the clitoris

1.26. The pudendal nerve:

A. Arises from the anterior primary rami of the second, third and fourth sacral nerves
B. Leaves the pelvis through the upper part of the greater sciatic foramen
C. Crosses the spine of the ischium on the medial side of the pudendal artery
D. Re-enters the pelvis through the lesser sciatic foramen
E. Enters the pudendal canal on the lateral side of the ischio-rectal fossa

Answers overleaf

1.24. A, D.

The levator ani is supplied by the fourth sacral nerve and by a branch which arises from the inferior haemorrhoidal (rectal) nerve or from the perineal division of the pudendal nerve. The obturator nerve arises from the second, third and fourth lumbar nerves. The pudendal nerve arises from the second, third and fourth sacral nerves.

1.25. A, C, E.

The pelvic splanchnic nerves arise from the anterior primary rami of the second and third (and fourth) sacral nerves. Visceromotor fibres are supplied to the detrusor muscle of the bladder and inhibiting fibres to its sphincter.

1.26. A, C, D, E.

The pudendal nerve leaves the pelvis through the lower part of the sciatic notch.

1.27. The sympathetic nervous system supplies:

A. Dilator fibres to the bronchial tree
B. Constrictor fibres to the coronary arteries
C. Constrictor fibres to the ciliary muscle of the eyes
D. Inhibitory fibres to the detrusor muscle of the bladder
E. Constrictor fibres to the muscles of the small intestine

1.28. The conduction system of the normal heart:

A. The cardiac impulse originates in the atrio-ventricular (A-V) node
B. The A-V node is situated in the wall of the coronary sinus
C. The impulse spreads by continuity between atrial and ventricular muscle
D. The A-V bundle lies in the intraventricular septum
E. The A-V bundle branches to supply each ventricle

1.29. The non-lactating adult human female breast:

A. Has a predominance of glandular tissue
B. Contains alveolar central cells which have undergone fatty degeneration
C. After menstruation there is periglandular infiltration of leucocytes
D. Has alveoli which are formed by small granular polyhedral cells
E. Is an example of an exocrine gland

Answers overleaf

1.27. A, D.

Local control via metabolites and hypoxia seems to be the main determinant of coronary flow. It is difficult to separate coronary vasoconstrictor or dilator sympathetic effects since sympathectomy does not increase coronary blood flow. Dilator fibres are supplied to the eyes and the muscles of the small intestine.

1.28. D, E.

The cardiac impulse originates in the sino-atrial (SA) node. The AV node is located in the right posterior portion of the interatrial septum. It is generally maintained that there is no specialized (nodal or Purkinje) pathway connecting the two nodes and that there are no Purkinje fibres in the atrial nodes.

1.29. C, D, E.

The main bulk of the breast is due to abundant fat surrounding the glandular tissue. The non-lactating alveoli are solid, more or less spherical masses of granular polyhydral cells which are potential alveoli. There is no suggestion of degeneration of the cells even after lactation has ceased. The glandular tissue returns to a 'resting' condition, any milk remaining is absorbed and the alveoli shrink, many losing their lumen.

1.30. The female breast:

A. Enlarges at puberty due to proliferation of ductal elements
B. Has ducts whose outer coats consist of longitudinal and transverse elastic fibres
C. Functions as a holocrine gland
D. During pregnancy undergoes fatty degeneration in the peripheral alveolar cells
E. Has abundant fatty tissue beneath the areola

1.31. The human female mammary gland:

A. Has alveoli which are mesodermal structures
B. Has 40–50 lobules
C. Starts to develop before the menarche
D. Can only reach full functional development as a result of pregnancy
E. Is innervated by branches derived from the fourth, fifth and sixth thoracic nerves

1.32. The thyroid gland:

A. Is related to the cartilages of the larynx
B. Does not move on swallowing
C. May be situated at the back of the tongue
D. Stores thyroglobulin
E. Forms thyroxine

Answers overleaf

1.30. A, B.

Holocrine glands are those which disintegrate to liberate the secretion e.g. sebaceous glands. The mammary gland functions as an aprocrine gland. That is one where the luminal part of the cell disintegrates to liberate its secretion leaving the nucleus and basal portion from which the cell regenerates to produce further secretion. Histocytes phagocytose the small amount of fat present in the alveoli secretion in the latter part of the pregnancy. There is no fat beneath the skin of the areola and nipple.

1.31. C, E.

The epithelial lining of its ducts is derived from the ectoderm, its supporting connective tissue from the mesenchyme. It consists of 15 to 20 lobules. The secreting activity of the cells lining the alveoli increases progressively during the latter half of pregnancy. True milk secretion commences a few days after parturition.

1.32. A, C, D, E.

The thyroid gland moves on swallowing.

1.33. The human pituitary gland:

A. Is situated in the posterior cranial fossa
B. Derives its blood supply from the circulus arteriosus (the circle of Willis)
C. Is directly related to the ninth (glosso-pharyngeal) cranial nerve
D. Is dependent for its proper function on neural and vascular connections with the hypothalamus
E. Contains pituicytes in the anterior lobe

1.34. In the pituitary gland:

A. The anterior lobe is the pars nervosa
B. Capillary blood passes from the adenohypophysis to the median eminence
C. The eosinophil cells produce growth hormone
D. The basophil cells produce oxytocin
E. Vasopressin is secreted by the posterior lobe

1.35. The pituitary gland:

A. Produces vasopressin
B. Has neural connections with the pineal body
C. Is entirely ectodermal in origin
D. Has a portal circulation
E. Has independent vascular systems for the anterior and posterior lobes

Answers overleaf

1.33. B, D.

The pituitary gland lies in the hypophyseal fossa of the sphenoid bone. It is not directly related to the glosso-pharyngeal nerve. The pituicytes are cells which are peculiar to the posterior lobe.

1.34. C, E.

The pars nervosa is the posterior lobe. Blood passes from the median eminence to the adenohypophysis. Oxytocin is produced from the posterior lobe.

1.35. C, D, E.

Vasopressin is hypothalmic in origin and stored in the posterior pituitary lobe. There are no neural connections with pineal body.

1.36. The hypothalamus:

A. Is responsible for temperature regulation
B. Forms part of the roof of the third ventricle
C. Contains the tuber cinereum
D. Contains the pulvinar
E. Influences parasympathetic activity via the lateral hypothalamic nucleus

1.37. The hypothalamus:

A. Forms part of the mid-brain
B. Is closely related to the optic tracts
C. Exerts specific actions by means of releasing factors
D. Is influenced by endocrine gland secretions
E. Has nerve connections with the anterior lobe of the pituitary gland

1.38. The adult spinal cord:

A. Extends to the middle of the sacrum
B. Is ensheathed in three protective membranes
C. Has no central canal
D. Is composed entirely of grey matter
E. Has a spinal ganglion in each dorsal nerve root

Answers overleaf

1.36. A, C, E.

The hypothalamus forms part of the floor of the third ventricle. The pulvinar occupies the whole breadth of the posterior quarter of the thalamus and constitutes its most posterior portion.

1.37. B, C, D.

The hypothalamus forms part of the fore-brain. The hypothalamus regulates the activity of the anterior pituitary through the release of factors which are carried by veins of the pituitary stalk.

1.38. B, E.

It only extends to the lower border of the first lumbar vertebrae or upper border of the second. It has a central canal and is composed of both grey and white matter.

2. EMBRYOLOGY, EARLY DEVELOPMENT OF THE FETUS AND THE FETAL CIRCULATION

2.1. Embryology:

A. Endodermal elements are involved in vaginal development

B. The ureter arises as an upgrowth from the lower part of the mesonephric duct

C. The coelomic epithelium of the ovary is the origin of the primitive germ cells

D. The labia minora arise from paired genital swellings

E. The phallic portion of the uro-genital sinus gives rise to the female urethra

2.2. In human gametogenesis and early development:

A. Maturation of spermatogonia to spermatozoa in man takes between 3–4 weeks

B. Embedding of the zygote usually occurs on the sixth day after fertilization

C. The second stage of meiosis is necessary before penetration of the sperm can occur

D. Embedding of the zygote occurs at the morula stage of development

E. The number of germ cells present in the ovary is greatest at about the fifth month of fetal life

2.3. In the formation and descent of the gonads:

A. Primordial germ cells are formed by the differentiation of the mesenchyme of the genital ridge

B. The gubernaculum of the testis is a derivative of the mesonephric duct

C. A diverticulum of the coelomic cavity extends into the mesenchyme of the gubernaculum of the testis to form the processus vaginalis

D. The ovary retains its intra-abdominal position because the gubernaculum of the ovary fails to reach the inguinal region

E. The homologues of the gubernaculum of the testis in the female include the ligament of the ovary

Answers overleaf

2.1. A, B.

The precise origin of the germ cells is still uncertain but comparative embryological evidence strongly suggests that they are derived either from the primitive endoderm or from a stem cell common to them and to the primitive endodermal cells.

The genital swellings remain separate as the labia majora and the genital folds also remain ununited forming the labia minora. In the female the whole of the urethra is derived from the vesico-urethral portion of the cloaca.

2.2. B, E.

Maturation of spermatogonia to spermatozoa takes about sixty to seventy-five days. The second meiotic division is not normally complete until penetration of the sperm. Embedding of the zygote occurs at the blastocyst stage.

2.3. C, E.

Cords of cells proliferate from the thickened coelonic epithelium forming sex cords and these extend into the underlying mesenchyme. Cells of a special kind appear in the genital ridges. They are the primordial germ cells and are generally believed to have migrated by way of the mesentery from a restricted area of the yolk sac wall close to the allantoic diverticulum.

Thus the gonads of both sexes are derived from three basic components, the coelomic epithelium, the mesenchyme of the adjacent part of the genital ridge and the primordial germ cells.

The testes at the seventh week of intrauterine life are attached to the posterior wall by the urogenital mesentery. The whole column of mesenchyme extending from the lower pole of the testis to the genital fold constitutes the gubernaculum testis.

The continuation of the gubernaculum of the ovary is the round ligament which does reach the inguinal region.

2.4. Development of the female genital tract:

A. The ovarian ligament is a derivative of the paramesonephric duct
B. The urogenital sinus receives the mesonephric ducts
C. The urogenital sinus is continuous with the allantois
D. The perineal body develops at the lower margin of the urorectal septum
E. The lower third of the vagina is derived from the mesonephric ducts

2.5. By the seventh week after fertilization the human embryo:

A. Is 14–16 cm long (crown-rump length)
B. Has an umbilical hernia
C. Has rudimentary digits
D. Heart has not yet started to beat
E. Mesonephric ducts have opened into the cloaca

2.6. During human embryogenesis:

A. The naso-labial folds and fronto-nasal processes are fused in embryos aged approximately 32 days (crown-rump length 5 mm)
B. The fetal sex can be identified by inspection of the external genitalia in embryos aged approximately 48 days (crown-rump length 20 mm)
C. Pigment appears in the optic vesicle in embryos aged approximately 36 days (crown-rump length 10 mm)
D. The circulation of blood commences by the beginning of the fourth week of life (7-somite stage)
E. The neural tube is normally completely closed in embryos aged approximately 52 days (crown-rump length 25 mm)

Answers overleaf

2.4. B, C, D.

The ovarian ligament is a derivative of the mesonephric fold. The lower part of the vagina is derived from sinovaginal bulb. The upper part is derived from the fused paramesonephric ducts.

2.5. A, B, C, E.

The heart has started to beat by the seventh week after fertilization.

2.6. C, D, E.

A difficult question but knowledge which may be relevant to the potential sites of teratogenic drugs.

In the six weeks after fertilization fusion of the naso-labial folds and fronto-nasal processes begins and the crown-rump length would be at least 10 mm.

The external genitalia are present and *may* show sexual differences by the end of the seventh week when the crown-rump length would be approaching 25–30 mm but are not readily identified by inspection.

2.7. The femur:

A. Begins to ossify during the seventh week of intra-uterine life
B. Grows in length mainly from the lower epiphyseal cartilage
C. Is ossified from three centres
D. Has cartilaginous extremities at birth
E. Is completely ossified before sexual maturity

2.8. In the normal fetus:

A. There is no ossification centre before the twelfth week of pregnancy
B. Each lumbar vertebra ossifies from three primary centres
C. Ossification centres in the calcaneus and in the talus are present by the thirty-second week of pregnancy
D. The primary centres for the ilium, ischium and pubic bones are generally fused at forty weeks
E. The ossification centre in the upper epiphysis of the tibia is usually present at forty weeks

2.9. The fetal and neonatal circulation:

A. In the fetal circulation the oxygen saturation of blood in the ductus arteriosus is greater than in the ductus venosus
B. In the fetal circulation oxygen tension in the descending aorta is less than in the aortic arch
C. After birth closure of the foramen ovale is due to a reversal of the pressure gradient between the right and left atria
D. Reversal or cessation of blood flow through the ductus arteriosus is aided by the increase in pulmonary arterial pressure which occurs at birth
E. Fetal blood can pass from the vena cava to the aorta without passing through the left atrium or left ventricle

Answers overleaf

2.7. A, B, D.

The femur is ossified from 5 centres. One each for the shaft, head, greater trochanter, lesser trochanter and lower end. Complete ossification does not take place until the late teens.

2.8. C, E.

Several centres of ossification of bone appear before the twelfth week. The lumbar vertebrae have two additional ossification centres for the mamillary processes. It is one of the exceptions from the usual three centres of ossification for vertebrae. At birth the three bones of the hip bone remain cartilaginous.

2.9. B, C, E.

The oxygen saturation of blood in the umbilical vein is believed to be about 80% compared with 98% saturation in the arterial circulation of the mother. The ductus venosus directs some of this blood directly to the vena cava and the remainder is mixed with the portal blood of the fetus. The portal and systemic blood of the fetus is only 25% saturated so that the inferior vena cava blood is approximately 65–70% saturated. Therefore the blood in the ductus arteriosus must be less than that in the ductus venosus.

The direction of flow in the ductus arteriosis is reversed due to a rise in the systemic vascular resistance resulting from exclusion of the placental circulation and a fall in the pulmonary resistance with expansion of the lungs.

Obliteration of the ductus arteriosis is also essential and this channel contracts rapidly at birth.

2.10. The fetal circulation:

- **A.** The ductus arteriosus is the dorsal proportion of the right sixth pulmonary aortic arch
- **B.** The septum secundum contains no foramen
- **C.** The umbilical vein drains into the ductus venosus
- **D.** The obliterated part of the hypogastric artery becomes the ligamentum teres of the adult
- **E.** The foramen ovale allows communication between the two ventricular cavities

2.11. The fetal circulation:

- **A.** Blood in the right atrium passes directly to the right ventricle
- **B.** Blood passes directly from the pulmonary trunk to the aorta
- **C.** Blood travels from the placenta in the umbilical arteries
- **D.** Blood in the right atrium passes directly to the left atrium
- **E.** The pressure in the left atrium is higher than that in the right atrium

2.12. The ductus venosus:

- **A.** Connects the left branch of the portal hepatic vein to the umbilical vein
- **B.** Conveys blood to the inferior vena cava before birth
- **C.** After birth becomes the ligamentum teres of the liver
- **D.** Becomes the lateral umbilical ligament of the adult
- **E.** Runs between the attached layers of the lesser omentum

Answers overleaf

2.10. C.

The ductus arteriosis is the dorsal portion of the *left* sixth (pulmonary) aortic arch.

The septum secundum has a foramen so that the septum primum can act as a flap like valve between the two atria.

The obliterated part of the hypogastric arteries are converted into fibrous cords which lie in the extra peritoneal fatty tissue of the abdominal wall and produce the medial umbilical folds of peritoneum.

The foramen ovale allows communication between the two atria.

2.11. A, B, D.

Blood from the placenta travels via the umbilical vein and returns to the placenta via the umbilical arteries. The pressure in the left atrium and right atrium is equal.

2.12. B, E.

The ductus venosus connects the definitive (left) umbilical vein with the right hepatocardiac vein. After birth the fibrous remnant of the umbilical vein persists as the ligamentum teres. The ductus venosus also fibroses after birth but remains as the ligamentum venosum joining the upper end of the ligamentum teres to the inferior vena cava.

2.13. The first maturation division of the primary oöcyte results in:

A. The haploid number of chromosomes
B. Two cells of equal size
C. Secondary oöcyte and first polar body
D. The formation of the oötid
E. Transformation due to the introduction of new deoxyribonucleic acid (DNA) molecules into the cell

2.14. Development of germ cells in the ovaries has the following feature:

A. Oögonia are formed until the time of puberty
B. A marked reduction in the number of oöcytes occurs between birth and puberty
C. All primary oöcytes enter the first meiotic prophase during fetal development before birth.
D. The second meiotic division is completed in all secondary oöcytes prior to ovulation
E. The genetic structure of the chromosomes in a secondary oöcyte is identical with that of the corresponding chromosomes in the primary oöcyte

2.15. Human spermatozoa:

A. Are formed in response to follicle stimulating hormone
B. Are developed from Sertoli cells
C. Are capable of fertilizing an oöcyte when taken from the seminiferous tubule
D. When mature have undergone a reduction division of their nucleus
E. Take 20–25 days to mature.

Answers overleaf

2.13. C.

In the first maturation division there is no reduction division and the cells produced are not of equal size. Whilst there is a spermatid there is no cell called oötid. From the primordial germ cell in the female and the ovum, three polar bodies are developed and in the male four spermatids, which later develop into spermatozoa.

In the first maturation division, there is an introduction of RNA rather than DNA.

2.14. B, C.

Oögonia undergo mitotic multiplication during the first six to seven months of intra-uterine life.

The second meiotic division is not normally completed until the oöcyte is penetrated by a spermatozoon.

The genetic structure in the primary and secondary oöcyte is different. One is diploid and the other haploid and therefore cannot be identical.

2.15. A, D.

Spermatozoa are formed from the primitive germ cells which line the seminiferous tubules. The sperms bury their heads in the Sertoli cells which are glycogen containing cells in the tubules from which the sperms apparently obtain nourishment. In man it takes about sixty-five to seventy-five days to form a mature sperm from a primitive germ cell. At the time when they leave the testis the spermatozoa are neither mobile nor fertile. They acquire both these properties during the passage within the epididymis.

In several mammalian species spermatozoa freshly deposited in the female are incapable of fertilizing the ovum, they require a period of time in the female reproductive tract in order to undergo 'capacitation'.

2.16. The human spermatozoon:

A. Is about 50 mμ in length
B. Consists largely of deoxyribonucleoprotein
C. Contains hyaluronidase in the acrosome
D. Contains adenosine triphosphate in the tail
E. Is motile when it leaves the testis

2.17. In early pregnancy:

A. The chorion laeve is the precursor of the true placenta
B. The uterine cavity is obliterated when the decidua capsularis comes in contact with the decidua vera
C. The syncytiotrophoblast is in contact with maternal blood
D. Both vitelline veins become the umbilical veins
E. The zygote begins to embed in the uterus at the age of three days

2.18. Trophoblast:

A. Develops from the blastocyst
B. Secretes gonadotrophins
C. Is physiologically invasive
D. Is primarily responsible for decidual formation
E. Forms part of the chorion

Answers overleaf

2.16. A, B, C, D.

The spermatozoa are not motile when they leave the testis they acquire this property during their passage in the epididymis.

2.17. B, C.

The chorion laeve becomes almost avascular and is opposite the area of the true placenta.

The principle visceral veins of the embryo are the two vitelline veins bringing blood from the yolk sac and the two umbilical veins returning blood from the placenta. With the decline in the yolk sac circulation the vitelline veins form the portal vein and its branches, the liver sinusoids, the hepatic veins and the uppermost part of the inferior vena cava.

By 6–6½ days following fertilization the fully developed blastocyst becomes attached to the uterine mucosa.

2.18. A, B, C, E.

The endometrial change to decidua formation is primarily dependent on the increased amounts of hormones produced by the corpus luteum of pregnancy.

2.19. In the placenta during the last trimester of pregnancy:

A. The cytotrophoblast has disappeared
B. The chorionic villi contain smooth muscle fibres
C. The intervillous space is sub-divided by septa
D. The trophoblast is separated from the fetal capillaries by a basement membrane
E. Non-myelinated nerve fibres are present

2.20. The human placenta:

A. Secretes chorionic gonadotrophin from the trophoblast
B. Has a negligible oxygen requirement
C. Is impermeable to substances with a molecular weight above 1000
D. Is able to synthesize oestrogens from acetate radicals
E. Transfers drugs from mother to fetus at a rate which depends only upon their lipid solubility

2.21. The amniotic fluid:

A. Is isotonic with maternal serum throughout pregnancy
B. Does not contain protein
C. At thirty-eight weeks of pregnancy, has an urea concentration exceeding that of maternal serum
D. Has a volume which is related to the period of gestation
E. Contains lecithin

Answers overleaf

2.19. B, C, D.

During the last trimester of pregnancy cytotrophoblast is still present. Non-myelinated fibres are not present.

2.20. A, C.

The placenta and fetus work together as a unit and it is estimated that both require about 16 mls oxygen per minute, which means a circulation of 300–400 mls blood per minute. This is less than most estimates of uterine blood flow at term of about 500–600 mls per minute.

The placenta has a limited role in steroid production. It requires precursors such as dehydroepiandrosterone or androsternedione from the fetal and maternal adrenals. It can convert these precursors by enzymes present in the placenta to oestrione and oestradiol 17β. The transfer of drugs varies considerably and depends on many factors such as their composition, size and structure.

2.21. C, D, E.

In the early stages of pregnancy, the amniotic fluid resembles plasma but as pregnancy advances, it becomes progressively more dilute. It contains some protein – the total concentration is about one twentieth of that in the serum.

2.22. The composition of human amniotic fluid varies as normal pregnancy advances in the following ways:

A. pH rises
B. Glucose concentration falls
C. Uric acid content rises
D. Oestriol concentration falls
E. Osmolality falls

2.23. In the full term baby on the second day of life:

A. The occipito-frontal circumference is 34–35 cm
B. The average concentration of blood sugar is over 100 mg per 100 ml (5.6 m.mol/l)
C. The blood volume is between 80–90 mls per kg body weight
D. Less than 40% of the haemoglobin is of the fetal type
E. The heart rate is 80–90 per minute

2.24. The following changes occur in the cardiovascular system at or shortly after birth:

A. The ductus venosus opens
B. Inferior vena caval pressure falls following occlusion of the umbilical cord
C. The ductus arteriosus is constricted
D. The pulmonary arterial pressure rises
E. The Hering-Breuer reflex operates only after the first breath

Answers overleaf

2.22. B, C, E.

The pH falls and the oestriol concentration rises.

2.23. A, C.

The average blood sugar is much lower than 100 mgms/100 ml (5.6 m.mol/1). At birth about 50% of the haemoglobin is of the fetal type and although it falls rapidly there would be little difference by the second day of life. The heart rate is over 100.

2.24. B, C.

The reverse is true for A and D. The Hering-Breuer reflex is present in the fetus.

3. GENETICS, CELL BIOLOGY AND EFFECTS OF RADIATION

3.1. The following diseases are sex linked:

A. Hereditary spherocytosis
B. Glucose-6-phosphate dehydrogenase deficiency
C. Factor IX deficiency (Christmas disease)
D. Haemoglobin C disease
E. Idiopathic thrombocytopenic purpura

3.2. An abnormal karyotype is characteristic of:

A. Phenylketonuria
B. Turner's syndrome (Gonadal dysgenesis)
C. Aplasia of the vagina
D. Congenital adrenogenital hyperplasia
E. Down's syndrome (Mongolism)

3.3. In the human cytogenetics:

A. Trisomic cells contain three pairs of a particular chromosome
B. Diploid cells contain homologous pairs of chromosomes
C. Chromosome homologues exchange portions of chromatids during mitotic prophase
D. Mature gametes are diploid cells
E. Haploid cells contain 23 chromosomes

Answers overleaf

3.1. B, C.

Glucose-6-phosphate dehydrogenase deficiency and Christmas disease are the only sex linked diseases of those given.

3.2. B, E.

Abnormal karyotypes are characteristically in gonadol dysgenesis and mongolism and not a feature of the other conditions given.

3.3. B, E.

Autosome trisomy means an additional chromosome. Chromatids begin to separate in the anaphase having lined up in equatorial plane in the metaphase. Mature gametes are haploid cells.

3.4. In Down's syndrome (Mongolism) of the G 21 trisomy type:

A. The paternal chromosomal pattern is normal
B. The maternal chromosomal pattern is normal
C. The total chromosome count is forty-six
D. Translocation G 21/22 is not found
E. Exfoliated fetal cells may demonstrate the chromosomal abnormality

3.5. In cell biology:

A. The principal constituent of chromosomes is deoxyribonucleic acid (DNA)
B. The active X chromosome in a female forms the chromatin (Barr) body
C. Acrocentric chromosomes are abnormal
D. Mosaicism is a result of non-disjunction during mitosis
E. Isochromosomes contain equal amounts of genetic material

3.6. In cytogenetics:

A. Normal secondary oöcytes have a diploid number of chromosomes
B. Sex (nuclear) chromatin is formed as a result of delay in ribonucleic acid (RNA)
C. Sex (nuclear) chromatin does not appear in fetal female cells until the twelfth week of gestation
D. A buccal smear from a normal male contains sex (nuclear) chromatin in more than 30% of nuclei
E. A cause of mosaicism is non-disjunction

Answers overleaf

3.4. A, B, D, E.

There are forty-seven chromosomes in Down's syndrome of the G 21 trisomy type.

3.5. A, D.

One X chromosome replicates later than its partner. This X chromosome is believed to be absent in the male and to form the sex chromatin (Barr Body) of the female interphase nucleus.

Acrocentric chromosomes are not abnormal.

Isochromosomes do not contain equal amounts of genetic material.

3.6. E.

Secondary oöcytes have a haploid number of chromosomes. Sex chromatin is formed as a result of delay in deoxyribonucleic acid (DNA) synthesis.

Sex determination occurs at the instant of conception.

Normal females have 40–70% of cells with a single sex chromatin body whilst normal males have none.

3.7. For the cytologist, previous irradiation of the cervix:

A. Increases the nuclear/cytoplasmic ratio in any malignant cells
B. Produces characteristic nucleolar halos
C. Decreases the size of the cells of any malignant cells
D. Increases the frequency of nuclear degeneration
E. Makes the interpretation of smears difficult

3.8. In radiotherapy:

A. ^{60}Co (cobalt) can be used as an irradiation source in place of radium
B. Radium is not used because it is too expensive
C. Low dose-rate treatments produce excellent clinical results
D. ^{137}Caesium is a byproduct of nuclear fission
E. Gamma rays from Caesium are more effective than x-rays of the same energy

3.9. Ionizing radiations:

A. With high energy external irradiation approximately 25% of the energy is lost by passing through the skin
B. The linear accelerator (4 MeV) can achieve effective penetration to a depth of 10 centimetres (4 inches) in human tissue
C. A large part of the energy of diagnostic x-rays is absorbed by bone
D. An isodose curve is a quantitative measure relating dose to depth of irradiation
E. Radiotherapy is more effective at temperatures below 36°C

Answers overleaf

3.7. A, C, D, E.

These are basic facts and there are no characteristic nucleolar changes.

3.8. A, C, D.

Radium is not used because it produces strong gamma rays and a radioactive gas as a daughter product. Both types of radiation are equally effective if they are of the same energy.

3.9. B, C, D.

Virtually no energy is lost when a megavoltage beam is passing through the skin. If temperatures are increased radiation can be more effective.

3.10. The effects of ionizing radiation on normal tissues:

A. The mucosa of the small bowel is one of the most radiosensitive tissues in the abdominal cavity
B. Small blood vessels are unaffected by radiation
C. Radiotherapy is usually given in divided doses so that normal tissues have time to recover partially between each dose
D. Bone damage is not seen with megavoltage radiation therapy
E. Damage is expressed preferentially in rapidly dividing cells

3.11. Radiation damage to tissue:

A. Is least in tissues with a high mitotic index
B. Is enhanced by hyperbaric oxygen
C. May be enhanced by previous treatment with chemotherapy
D. Does not cause neoplasia
E. May cause visible chromosomal damage in circulating lymphocytes

Answers overleaf

3.10. A, C, E.

Radiation damage of small arteries is responsible for the late tissue damage seen after ionising radiation. Bone damage is less common with megavoltage radiation therapy but is a function of dose.

3.11. B, C, E.

Damage is greatest in tissues with a high mitotic index. Leukaemias and solid tumours are well recognised complications of exposure to ionising radiation.

4. MICROBIOLOGY AND IMMUNOLOGY

4.1. The gonococcus:

A. Is a gram positive diplococcus
B. Grows readily in culture on ordinary nutrient Agar
C. Will grow in culture at temperatures under 34°C
D. Is unable to penetrate stratified squamous epithelium
E. Causes an inflammatory response by production of a gonococcal endotoxin

4.2. The causative organism of:

A. Condyloma lata is Neisseria gonorrhoeae
B. Chancroid is Haemophilus ducreyi
C. Granuloma inguinale is Donovania granulomatis (Calymmatobacterium granulomatis)
D. Primary chancre is Treponema pertenue
E. Yaws is Haemophilus vaginalis

4.3. Candida albicans:

A. Gives a positive reaction to Gram's stain
B. Is an anaerobic organism
C. Is associated with diabetes mellitus
D. Is characterised by flagella
E. Is inhibited by oral tetracycline therapy

Answers overleaf

4.1. D, E.

The gonococcus is a gram negative organism and will not grow on nutrient agar. It also has a relatively narrow temperature range for growth.

4.2. B, C.

Neisseria gonorrhoeae causes gonorrhoea whilst condylomata lata are found in the secondary stage of syphillis. Yaws is due to infection with Treponema pertenue whereas the primary chancre is due to treponema pallidum.

4.3. A, C.

This yeast like fungus is strongly Gram positive has pseudohypae (not flagella) and is aerobic. Whilst the association of alimentary and vaginal infection during and after broad spectrum antibiotics is well known, it is in practice, often neglected.

4.4. Organisms associated with infection of the female urinary tract are:

A. Escherichia coli
B. Mycobacterium tuberculosis
C. Döderlein's bacillus
D. Staphylococcus pyogenes
E. Proteus mirabilis

4.5. Vesical schistosomiasis:

A. Is acquired by eating snails
B. Causes intermittent haematuria
C. Is diagnosed by finding schistosoma haematobium eggs in the urine
D. Is endemic in the Caribbean area
E. Is sexually transmitted

4.6. The following organisms are known to be responsible for food poisoning:

A. Staphylococcus aureus
B. Streptococcus pyogenes
C. Salmonella typhimurium
D. Klebsiella aerogenes
E. Clostridium botulinum

Answers overleaf

4.4. A, B, D, E.

Döderleins bacilli have a protective function in the adult genital tract because they form a lactic acid from the glycogen of the epithelium and thereby keep the vaginal secretion too acid for most other organisms. The other organisms are all potentially pathogenic in the urinary tract.

4.5. B, C.

The parasites of Schistosoma (Bilharzia) are dioecious trematodes which depend on certain varieties of fresh water snails as intermediate hosts. The forked-tail cercarie leave the snails, swim freely in water and penetrate the skin of man. The schistosomes live in the mesenteric and pelvic veins. The female deposits her eggs in small vessels, whence they penetrate gradually into the intestines and bladder and pass out in the urine and faeces. Schistosoma haematobin causes above all, inflammation of the urogenital system, bloody urine (papilloma formation), fistula and malignant tumours.

S. Mansome is endemic in the Caribbean area (West Indies) whereas S. haematobium is more common in Africa.

4.6. A, C, E.

The most important food pathogens are the salmonella, Staph. pyogenes, Cl. welchii and Cl. botulinum.

4.7. Examination of a stained deposit of cerebro-spinal fluid from a case of meningitis reveals Gram-negative intracellular diplococci. These are likely to be:

A. Diplococcus pneumoniae (pneumococcus)
B. Haemophilus influenzae
C. Neisseria gonorrhoeae (gonococcus)
D. Neisseria meningitidis (meningococcus)
E. Staphylococcus aureus (pyogenes)

4.8. Leucocytosis characteristically follows infection by:

A. Staphylococcus pyogenes
B. Streptococcus pyogenes
C. Escherichia coli
D. Meningococci
E. Brucella melitensis

4.9. Bacterial sterilisation:

A. Dry heat is more effective than moist heat
B. Milk is sterilised by the process of pasteurization
C. Vegatative bacteria are more readily killed than bacterial spores
D. The presence of protein increases the resistance of bacteria to heat
E. Moist heat is most effective at a neutral pH

Answers overleaf

4.7. D.

Pneumococci are Gram positive diplococci. Haemophilus influenzae are Gram negative but not diplococci. The gonococcus does not cause meningitis. Staph. pyogenes are not diplococci and are Gram positive.

4.8. A, B, C, D.

Leucocytosis is characteristic of a pyogenic infection. Brucella melitensis is primarily a pathogen of goats. Infections with brucellosis in man is primarily a disease of the reticulo-endothelial system. Acute infections with brucellosis may be associated with a daily or diurnal remitting fever.

4.9. C, D.

Bacteria are intrinsically more susceptible to moist heat than to dry heat. Most vegetative bacteria are killed by exposure under moist conditions, to temperatures of 60 to 65° C for half an hour. Hence the pasteurization of milk. Spores will withstand boiling for a considerable time and boiling would be regarded as inadequate for the sterilisation.

The term 'sterilisation' means the killing or removal of all micro-organisms including spores. Hence the importance of washing instruments before sterilisation. Most bacteria will only grow in the pH range 5–9 and the growth of many bacteria is sharply restricted to the neighbourhood of pH 7.

4.10. Endotoxins:

A. Are derived from Gram-negative bacteria
B. Have a specific action
C. Are more toxic than exotoxins
D. Are neutralised by their homologous antitoxin
E. Can be toxoided

4.11. Passive immunity is conferred by:

A. Precipitated toxoid
B. Formalised toxoid
C. Antitoxic serum
D. Convalescent serum
E. Live vaccine

4.12. The following examples are of a disease correctly coupled with a serological test:

A. Lymphopathia venereum – Frei test
B. Myeloid leukaemia – Complement fixation test
C. Infectious mononucleosis – Nagler reaction
D. Syphilis – Khan test
E. Neonatal jaundice – Widal reaction

Answers overleaf

4.10. A.

Endotoxins are released when bacteria die and are mainly associated with gram negative organisms. They are complex lipopolysaccharides and are relatively heat stable. Their toxic effects, which are widespread, depend little upon the species from which the toxins are derived. Weight for weight, endotoxins are less potent than exotoxins. Endotoxins are little if at all antigenic.

4.11. C, D.

Toxoids and live vaccines are used for active immunisation.

4.12. A, D.

Complement absorbs specifically to antigen-antibody complexes and consequently fixation of complement can be used as an indicator that an antigen-antibody combination has occurred. Complement fixation is on the whole the most useful technique for the estimation of anti-viral antibody.

The Nagler reaction is used for the detection of Cl. welchii and can be recognised even in a mixed culture whilst the Paul-Bunnell test helps in the diagnosis of infectious mononucleosis.

The Widal reaction is a test for enteric fever and other Salmonella infections.

4.13. BCG inoculation:

- **A.** If positive produces a skin flare
- **B.** If positive results in regional node enlargement
- **C.** Should be given intramuscularly
- **D.** Uses live attenuated tubercle bacilli
- **E.** Is effective in the newborn

4.14. The following diseases are caused by infection with spirochaetes:

- **A.** Infectious mononucleosis
- **B.** Yaws
- **C.** Undulant fever
- **D.** Vincent's angina
- **E.** Granuloma inguinale

4.15 The incubation period of:

- **A.** Measles is 1–7 days
- **B.** Mumps is 1–7 days
- **C.** Diphtheria is 14–21 days
- **D.** Paratyphoid fever is 14–21 days
- **E.** Rubella is 14–21 days

Answers overleaf

4.13. B, D, E.

The Baccille Calmette Geurin (BCG) is bovine Myco. Tuberculosis strain attenuated by prolonged artificial culture. When injected into humans it causes only local lesions. The vaccine is given as a small intradermal injection of a suspension of the live baccilli. A small tuberculous ulcer develops a few weeks after vaccination and persists for several months before it heals leaving a small scar.

4.14. B, D.

Infectious mononucleosis is a viral infection. Undulant fever is a brucellosis infection and granuloma inguinale is a chronic granulomatous venereal disease due to calymmatobacterium granulomatus.

4.15. E.

The incubation period of measles is 7–21 days (usually 10–11); mumps is 12–26 days (average 18); diphtheria is 1–6 days (average 2); paratyphoid is 6–15 (usually 10–12) and rubella is 14–21 (average 18).

4.16. Herpes zoster:

A. Is due to infection with the virus of herpes simplex
B. Is similar to chicken-pox (varicella) aetiologically
C. Recurs infrequently in the same patient
D. Is a premalignant condition
E. May be provoked by immunosuppressive drugs

4.17. Characteristically a virus:

A. Measures less than 200 mμ in diameter
B. Has a metabolic system of its own
C. Divides by binary fission
D. Is an obligatory intracellular parasite
E. Can synthesise new virus particles

4.18. Humoral antibodies in the human are:

A. Immunoglobulins
B. Not produced after removal of the thymus gland
C. Produced in response to soluble antigens
D. The main factor responsible for the allograft (homograft) reaction
E. The main immunological defence against acute infections

Answers overleaf

4.16. B, C, E.

The viruses of chicken pox and shingles (zoster) are indistinguishable from each other in the laboratory. The chicken-pox/shingles virus can be differentiated from herpes simplex virus by its failure to produce lesions on the chorio-allantoic membranes of eggs. Chicken pox is a mild disease and shingles a rare one. Childhood infection with chicken pox, whilst it commonly gives lifelong protection against that disease, does not prevent shingles. No drugs are known to be effective against the virus and disturbance of the host parasite relationship is disturbed by all immunosuppressive drug therapy.

4.17. A, D, E.

The human pathogenic viruses vary in size from the smallest, which are about 20 mμ in diameter to the larger viruses of the pox group which measure from 250 mμ to 300 mμ in their longest axis. Viruses are obligatory parasites and will only grow within living cells. They can only reproduce if they can make use of the metabolic machinery of the host cell for the production of the raw materials required for the synthesis of virus components. Viruses increase in number by replication.

4.18. A, C, E.

Removal of the thymus leads to a diminished response to new antigens.

It is considered that the mechanism of skin homograft rejection is similar to that operating in delayed cellular hypersensitivity reactions with the cellular immune reaction as the predominant factor.

4.19. Which of the following are examples of cell-mediated immune reactions:

A. The tuberculin reaction
B. Contact sensitivity to simple chemical substances
C. Asthma
D. The homograft reaction
E. Anaphylaxis

4.20. Human anaphylactic phenomena:

A. Depend upon the presence of appropriate reagins (IgE antibodies)
B. Are the result of antibody-antigen reactions which occur in the blood stream
C. Are often associated with histamine release
D. Are often associated with an eosinophil leucocytosis
E. In anaphylactic individuals desensitization depends upon the production of IgG antibodies

4.21. An allergic response in man may be characterised by:

A. Abnormal levels of immunoglobin E (IgE)
B. Liberation of histamine
C. Granular discharge from mast cells
D. Elevation of serum 5-hydroxytryptamine
E. Hypocalcaemia

Answers overleaf

4.19. A, B, D.

Asthma and anaphylaxis are examples of hypersensitivity reactions.

4.20. A, C, D, E.

The antibody antigen reaction in the blood stream is responsible for immunity. Anaphylactic hypersensitivity occurs in, or in association with, tissue cells.

4.21. A, B, C.

5-hydroxytryptamine (serotonin) is the main mediator of anaphylactic reactions in rats and mice, it does not appear to play any significant role in human anaphylactic syndromes. When the calcium iron concentration is low only the parathyroid gland is stimulated to release its hormone.

The main source of histamine is from the mast cells, the granules of which appear to be a loose complex of histamine and heparin.

4.22. ABO blood group antigens:

A. Are attached to the haemoglobin molecule
B. Contain mucopolysaccharides
C. Are determined by genes carried by sex chromosomes
D. Can be found in the saliva
E. Are present in red cell precursors

4.23. Fetal blood:

A. Fetal cells do not appear in the maternal blood stream before the twenty-eighth week of pregnancy
B. Fetal haemoglobin resists elution by an acid buffer
C. Fetal/maternal ABO compatibility protects against rhesus sensitisation
D. The quantity of bile pigments in the amniotic fluid reflects the severity of fetal haemolysis
E. A positive direct Coombs' test on the baby's red cells indicates the presence of maternal antibodies on the fetal cells

4.24. With respect to human blood groups:

A. Antigens on the surface of red cells are controlled directly by specific genes
B. The gene pairs for most blood antigens lie on the sex chromosomes
C. The 'naturally occurring' antibodies are IgM globulins
D. There are no antibodies (agglutinins) to the ABO group system in group O blood
E. 'Naturally occurring' blood group antibodies are incomplete antibodies

Answers overleaf

4.22. B, D, E.

The ABO group antigens are carried on the surface of the red blood cells. The antigen molecule has a chemical structure containing an amino-acid complex combined with a polysaccharide residue which usually confers specificity on the molecule. The antigens are genetically controlled by autosomes.

4.23. B, D, E.

Fetal cells can be detected in the maternal circulation before twenty-eight weeks e.g. following an abortion or amniocentesis, using the Kleihauer test. This test makes use of the fact that fetal haemoglobin is more resistant to an acid buffer than adult (maternal) haemoglobin. It is fetal-maternal *in*compatibility which provides a natural protection against rhesus sensitisation.

4.24. A, C.

The gene pairs are related to autosomes. There are agglutinins in the plasma (anti A and anri B). They are not incomplete antibodies.

5. PHARMACOLOGY

5.1. Chloramphenicol:

A. Contains a nitrobenzene group
B. Has a narrow spectrum of antibacterial activity
C. Is effective against gram negative organisms
D. Is metabolised in the liver
E. Can cause leucopenia

5.2. Streptomycin:

A. Is excreted actively by the renal tubules
B. Is primarily bacteriostatic
C. May cause 'drug fever'
D. Is destroyed by gastric juice if given by mouth
E. Is rapidly broken down by the liver

Answers overleaf

5.1. A, C, D, E.

Chloramphenicol has a wide range of activity against common organisms as well as salmonella and rickettsiae.

5.2. C.

Streptomycin is excreted unchanged by the kidney. If renal function is poor the drug will accumulate and cause serious toxicity. In therapeutic doses it is not broken down in the liver to any great extent. It is primarily bacteriocidal. Absorption is negligible and it can therefore be used to destroy intestinal bacteria. Since oral streptomycin may be used prior to bowel surgery and for dysentery it is not destroyed in the stomach.

5.3. Morphine

- **A.** Is metabolised in the liver
- **B.** Impairs conduction in sensory nerves
- **C.** Depresses the vomiting centre
- **D.** Constricts the pupils
- **E.** Stimulates release of vasopressin

5.4. Barbiturates:

- **A.** Depress the respiratory centre
- **B.** Inhibit the activity of certain liver enzyme systems
- **C.** Are usually metabolized in the liver
- **D.** Have anticonvulsant properties
- **E.** Are rapidly excreted in acid urine

5.5. Atropine given subcutaneously in therapeutic doses:

- **A.** Increases the resting heart rate
- **B.** Produces vasodilatation of the skin
- **C.** Reduces the flow of saliva
- **D.** Produces overactivity of the small intestine
- **E.** Is hypnotic

Answers overleaf

5.3. A, D, E.

Morphine sulphate does not affect conduction in sensory nerves and it stimulates the vomiting centre.

5.4. A, C, D.

Barbiturates have no effect on liver enzymes systems. The reason that there is little renal excretion of most barbiturates is not that they do not appear in the glomerular filtrate, but because if unionised they diffuse back into the circulation through the renal tubule. This diffusion will be less if the drug is ionised since barbiturates are weak organic acids. Ionisation will be maximal at a higher (alkaline) pH. Renal excretion of barbiturate can therefore be enhanced by making the urine alkaline to pH 8.

5.5. A, B, C.

The smooth muscle of the gastro-intestinal tract is relaxed by the atropine with reduction of tone and peristalsis. The central nervous system is stimulated by atropine.

5.6. Thiopentone given intravenously:

A. Is metabolised within minutes
B. Is excreted rapidly from the body
C. Has a high degree of protein binding
D. Has a high fat solubility
E. Is predominantly excreted in the urine

5.7. Halothane:

A. Is a bronchoconstrictor
B. Has a direct relaxant effect on uterine muscle
C. Is a volatile agent
D. Is inflammable
E. Lowers blood pressure in a direct relationship to the inspired concentration

5.8. The following drugs are hypotensive agents:

A. Benzothiadiazide diuretics
B. Rauwolfia alkaloids
C. Guanethidine
D. Hydrallazine
E. Ergometrine

Answers overleaf

5.6. C, D.

Thiopentone is metabolised slowly by the liver and other body tissues. The reason for its rapid action is its rapid distribution into the well perfused viscera and lean tissues of the body. For most barbiturates, including thiopentone, excretion is chiefly hepatic with little urinary excretion.

5.7. B, C, E.

Halothane is a bronchodilator and non-explosive as well as non-inflammable.

5.8. A, B, C, D.

Hypertension is a well documented adverse side effect of ergometrine.

5.9. A woman taking a monoamine oxidase inhibitor may become severely hypertensive after consuming foods or drinks which:

A. Contain synthetic preservatives
B. Have been cooked and then reheated
C. Contain milk protein
D. Are contaminated with bacterial toxins
E. Contain tea

5.10. The anticoagulant heparin:

A. Acts by blocking the action of fibrinogen
B. Is a polysaccharide
C. Crosses the placenta
D. Acts by blocking the action of thrombin
E. Has its action reversed by protamine sulphate

Answers overleaf

5.9. ALL FALSE

The following foods can produce or may be expected to be capable of producing dangerous hypersensitive effects. Cheese, especially if well matured, yogurt, some pickled herring, broad beans, yeast extracts, meat extracts (Bovril), wine and beer. This list is probably incomplete but none of the above are included in the items in question.

5.10. B, D, E.

Heparin in the presence of a plasma co-factor is mainly active as an antithrombin and antithromboplastin. It has a large molecule and does not cross the placenta.

5.11. The following biochemical changes are likely to be found in a woman who has received an oral contraceptive containing oestrogen and progestogen for several months:

A. An increase in blood concentration of serum alkaline phosphatase
B. An increase in the blood concentration of protein-bound iodine
C. An increase in the blood concentration of free thyroxine
D. An increase in the blood concentration of fibrinogen
E. A reduction in the plasma concentration of cortisol

5.12. The administration of oestrogens:

A. Increases the concentration in serum of thyroxine-binding globulin
B. Leads to water retention
C. Leads to a rise in the blood lipids
D. Reduces the amount of cortisol binding globulins
E. Alters glucose tolerance

5.13. Prostaglandin $F_{2\alpha}$ administered in a therapeutic dose will produce:

A. Water retention
B. Increased uterine contractility
C. Increased small bowel peristalsis
D. Dilatation of the bronchi
E. Elevation of the blood pressure

Answers overleaf

5.11. A, B, D.

The amount of thyroid binding globulin is elevated and as a result the free thyroxine is reduced. There is increase in plasma concentration of cortisol not a reduction.

5.12. A, B, E.

Blood lipids are usually reduced by oestrogens. Administration of oestrogens increases the amount of cortisol binding globulins.

5.13. B, C.

Unlike other oxytoxics prostaglandins do not cause water retention. According to circumstances the prostaglandin can cause smooth muscle to constrict or relax. Because of constriction of the bronchi, it is usually advised that caution should be used if the drug is contemplated being used in asthmatics. The relaxation of the smooth muscle of blood vessels would tend to lower blood pressure.

5.14. Cytotoxic agents:

- **A.** The nitrogen mustard group of drugs are antimetabolic agents
- **B.** Cyclophosphamide is an alkylating agent
- **C.** Methotrexate is an antimitotic agent
- **D.** Androgens have a beneficial effect in certain mammary gland cancers
- **E.** No antibiotic so far developed has a cytotoxic or cytostatic action

5.15. The administration of chloroquine phosphate may cause:

- **A.** Retinopathy
- **B.** Bleaching of hair
- **C.** Changes in the cornea
- **D.** Deafness
- **E.** Photosensitivity

5.16. The human fetus is adversely affected by:

- **A.** Cytomegalic inclusion disease
- **B.** ECHO virus
- **C.** Cephaloridine
- **D.** Streptomycin
- **E.** Heroin addiction of the mother

Answers overleaf

5.14. B, D.

The nitrogen mustards are alkylating agents and interact with DNA. Methotrexate is an antimetabolite and a folic acid antagonist. There are now several antibiotics which act on nuclear function in a variety of ways e.g. actinomycin C and D and therefore cytotoxic.

5.15. A, B, C.

Deafness and photosensitivity have not been reported following chloroquine administration.

5.16. A, D, E.

There is no evidence that the ECHO virus or cephaloridine adversely affects the fetus.

5.17. Drugs in pregnancy:

A. Digitalis does not cross the placenta
B. Hydrallazine causes contriction of placental vessels
C. Methotrexate does not cross the placenta
D. Heparin crosses the placenta
E. Hexamethonium crosses the placenta

5.18. The effect of drugs on the uterus:

A. Oestrogen encourages myometrial hypertrophy
B. Castor oil has a direct action on the uterus
C. Intravenous ethyl alcohol inhibits contraction of the pregnant uterus
D. Tubocurarine paralyses uterine muscle
E. Vasopressin stimulates uterine contractility

5.19. The prostaglandins:

A. Are saturated fatty acids
B. Are present in many mammalian tissues
C. Have been isolated from human amniotic fluid
D. Produce a different myometrial response at different stages of the menstrual cycle
E. Have identical physiological actions

Answers overleaf

5.17. E.

The correct answers are essentially the reverse of the indïvidual items.

Digitalis and methotrexate do cross the placenta and heparin does not.

Hydrallazine causes vasodilation of the placental vessels.

5.18. A, C, E.

Castor oil affects the smooth muscle of the intestine, the effect if any on the uterus would be indirect. Tubocurarine does not paralyse uterine muscle it produces a neuromuscular block by competition with acetylcholine.

5.19. B, C, D.

Prostaglandins are modified hydroxyacids derived from prostnoic acid and are unsaturated fatty acids. They can be synthesised. There are at least fourteen naturally occurring prostaglandins. Prostaglandins have many actions that differ according to the particular prostaglandin used and to the physiological state of that organ.

6. PATHOLOGY

6.1. Essential features of abscess formation are:

A. Eosinophil leucocytes
B. Destruction of tissue
C. Pyaemia
D. Septicaemia
E. Neutrophil leucocytes

6.2. Substances important in the increased vascular permeability of acute inflammation include:

A. Globulin permeability factor
B. Cortisol
C. Histamine
D. Plasma kinins
E. Serotonin

6.3. Phagocytosis is a characteristic function of the following types of cell:

A. Plasma cell
B. Polymorphonuclear leucocyte
C. Küpffer cell
D. Histiocyte
E. Melanocyte

Answers overleaf

6.1. B, E.

The essential features of an abscess are a lining pyogenic membrane which consists of necrotic tissue and a fibrinous exudate heavily infiltrated with polymorphonuclear leucocytes.

6.2. A, C, D, E.

Cortisol does not increase the vascular permeability in acute infection.

6.3. B, C, D.

Plasma cells and melanocytes do not possess phagocytosis as a characteristic feature.

6.4. Eosinophilia is characteristic of:

A. Diphtheria
B. Asthma
C. Infectious mononucleosis
D. Trichiniasis
E. Tuberculosis

6.5. Macrophages:

A. Produce antibody in response to antigenic stimulation
B. Are motile
C. Are phagocytic
D. Have lysosomes in their cytoplasm
E. Are derived from polymorphonuclear leucocytes

Answers overleaf

6.4. B, D.

Diphtheria is associated with a neutrophilia and miliary tuberculosis with a leucopenia. Infectious mononucleosis is associated with a lymphocytosis whose nuclear shape may resemble that of a monocyte but the chromatin lacks the typical features of a monocyte.

Eosinophilia is found in certain hypersensitivity states, e.g. asthma, hay fever and also chronic skin diseases, e.g. pemphigus. It also occurs with all helminthic infestations which invade tissues.

6.5. B, C, D.

The macrophages do not produce antibody and are not derived from polymorphonuclear leucocytes.

6.6. The inflammatory reaction varies with the casual organism. Which of the following pairs are correctly associated:

A. Staphylococcus aureus – spreading inflammation
B. Clostridium welchii – localised inflammation
C. Corynebacterium diphtheriae – pseudo-membrane formation
D. Streptococcus pyogenes – gas formation
E. Myobacterium tuberculosis – granulomatous inflammation

6.7. A typical tuberculous follicle contains:

A. Polymorphonuclear leucocytes
B. Lymphocytes
C. Epitheloid cells
D. Foreign body giant cells
E. Areas of haemorrhage

6.8. Cerebro-spinal fluid from an acute pyogenic meningitis would show:

A. An increased sugar content
B. An increased protein content
C. An increased cellular content
D. The presence of acid-fast bacilli
E. Blood or blood pigment

Answers overleaf

6.6. C, E.

The staphylococcus aureus is associated with a localised inflammation, the streptococcus pyogenes with spreading inflammation and clostridium welchii with gas formation.

6.7. B, C.

The tubercle follicle consists of a central mass of caseation surrounded by epithelioid and giant cells which in turn are enclosed in a wide zone of small round cells.

Polymorphonuclear leucocytes, foreign body giant cells and areas of haemorrhage are not present in a typical follicle.

6.8. B, C.

The protein content of CSF is raised in all types of meningitis (including viral). Blood sugar and chloride levels are reduced in all types of bacterial meningitis especially the tuberculous variety.

In an acute pyogenic meningitis acid fast bacilli and blood or blood pigment would be absent.

6.9. Granuloma is a type of inflammatory reaction characteristic of:

A. Tuberculosis
B. Rheumatoid arthritis
C. Regional ileitis
D. Staphylococcal pyaemia
E. Sarcoidosis

6.10. Characteristically, syphilitic arteritis:

A. Is found in the aortic arch
B. Is found in the descending aorta
C. Causes intimal ulceration
D. Causes fibrous scarring
E. Produces aortic valve incompetence

6.11. Ulceration of the bowel mucosa is characteristic of the following:

A. Diverticulosis coli
B. Coeliac disease
C. Tuberculous enteritis
D. Regional ileitis
E. Typhoid fever

Answers overleaf

6.9. A, B, C, E.

Granuloma occur in chronic inflammation which share a common characteristic in that the inflammatory lesions take a nodular or tumour like form. The term granuloma, though firmly established, is misleading. It implies a neoplasm of granulation tissue but the tumour is simply a swelling. While the granulation tissue is strikingly different from that of ordinary non-specific infection (e.g. staphylococcal).

6.10. A, D, E.

The abdominal aorta is rarely attacked in syphilis. The effects of syphilis are first noted in the tunica adventitia and spread inwards to the media where it destroys most of the elastic tissue. The intima is rarely affected.

6.11. C, D, E.

Ulceration is not a characteristic feature of diverticulosis or coeliac disease.

6.12. The following substances can be constituents of emboli:

- **A.** Fat
- **B.** Gas
- **C.** Neoplastic tissue
- **D.** Bacteria
- **E.** Trophoblastic cells

6.13. Embolism is a sequel to:

- **A.** Pelvic vein thrombosis
- **B.** Fracture of long bones
- **C.** Mitral stenosis
- **D.** Essential hypertension
- **E.** Administration of progestogens

6.14. The chief chemical constituents of urinary calculi are:

- **A.** Cholesterol
- **B.** Sodium chloride
- **C.** Uric acid
- **D.** Blood pigments
- **E.** Calcium phosphate

Answers overleaf

6.12. A, B, C, D, E.

6.13. A, B, C.

Embolism is not a sequel to essential hypertension or the administration of progestogens. Oestrogens have been shown to be associated with an increased incidence of thrombo-embolism.

6.14. C, E.

The common primary urinary calculi are urate stones composed of uric acid with sodium or potassium urate. Calcium oxalate stones, cystine stones and xanthine stones also occur, although the last two are rare.

Secondary calculi are composed of calcium phosphate and magnesium, ammonium phosphate together with a variable amount of calcium carbonate.

6.15. Haemochromatosis:

A. Is more common in females
B. Predisposes to diabetes mellitus
C. Is usually accompanied by a serum iron in excess of 2g per 100 ml
D. May be evoked by parenteral iron therapy given for the treatment of haemoglobinopathies
E. Predisposes to primary carcinoma of the liver

6.16. Deposition of iron pigment in the liver is a feature of:

A. Chronic haemolytic anaemia
B. Malignant melanoma
C. Carcinoid syndrome
D. Diabetes insipidus
E. Erythroblastosis fetalis

Answers overleaf

6.15. B, D, E.

Haemochromatosis most commonly affects men; women presumably being protected by their menstrual loss. The total iron binding capacity of the plasma is 300–360 μg per 100 ml and is normally about a third saturated with iron (the normal level is 60–200 μg per 100 ml). Although raised in haemochromatosis it is not raised to the excessive level given.

6.16. A, E.

An excess of iron deposition is seen when (i) there is overloading due to excessive absorption, e.g. when the normal regulating mechanism for iron absorption is impaired as in haemochromatosis. (ii) There is increased haemopoietic activity, e.g. chronic haemolytic anaemia especially thalassaemia, and (iii) when there is a great increase in the iron content of the diet.

Only A and E fit into the above criteria.

6.17. Haemolysis occurs in:

- **A.** Glucose 6-phosphate dehydrogenase deficiency in the newborn
- **B.** Plasmodium falciparum infection
- **C.** Clostridium welchii infection
- **D.** Diabetes
- **E.** Amyloidosis

6.18. In uncomplicated homozygous (β) thalassaemia there is:

- **A.** Hypochromasia
- **B.** Reduction in Haemoglobin A_2
- **C.** Increase in Haemoglobin F
- **D.** No depletion of iron stores
- **E.** Megaloblasts in bone marrow

6.19. Benign tumours are characterised by:

- **A.** Cellular pleomorphism
- **B.** Spontaneous regression
- **C.** Smallness in size
- **D.** Cellular differentiation
- **E.** Lymphocytic reaction

Answers overleaf

6.17. A, B, C.

Haemolysis does not occur in amyloidosis or diabetes, whether mellitus or insipidus.

6.18. A, C, D.

There is an increase in Hb A_2.
The blood film resembles a very severe iron deficiency anaemic picture and there will not be megaloblasts in the bone marrow.

6.19. D.

The only characteristic feature of a benign tumour listed is cellular differentiation. Both structurally and functionally the tumour cells tend to copy the parent tissue.

6.20. The following neoplasms are benign:

- **A.** Leiomyoma
- **B.** Chondroma
- **C.** Rhabdomyoma
- **D.** Seminoma
- **E.** Meningioma

6.21. Metaplasia is characterised by:

- **A.** An increase in the number and size of cells
- **B.** Variation in the size and shape of cells
- **C.** An increase in the nucleo-cytoplasmic ratio of cells
- **D.** Cloudy swelling of cells
- **E.** An acute inflammatory reaction

6.22. The following have carcinogenic properties:

- **A.** Sunlight
- **B.** Soot
- **C.** Asbestos
- **D.** Mineral oil
- **E.** X-rays

Answers overleaf

6.20. A, B, C, E.

The seminoma is a carcinoma of the testis derived from the seminiferous epithelium.

6.21. ALL FALSE

Metaplasia is a condition in which there is a change of one of differentiated tissue to another type of similarly differentiated tissue. None of the items would be covered by this definition.

6.22. A, B, C, D, E.

All the items given have carcinogenic properties.

6.23. Squamous cell carcinoma occurs as a primary neoplasm in:

A. Skin
B. Tongue
C. Colon
D. Oesophagus
E. Fallopian tube

6.24. A carcinoid tumour has the following characteristics:

A. Its cells have the ability to reduce silver salts
B. It may arise in an ovarian teratoma
C. It is a benign form of neoplasm
D. Patients with this tumour have chorionic gonadotrophin in their urine
E. It is associated with pulmonary hypertension

Answers overleaf

6.23. A, B, D.

Squamous cell carcinomas arise in any site normally covered by stratified squamous epithelium. Neither the colon or the Fallopian tube have squamous epithelium present.

6.24. A, B, E.

The tumour is locally invasive and may metastasize to the regional lymph nodes and the liver, especially in lesions of the small and large bowel.

In about 1% of all cases, and in 20% of those with metastases, an endocrine syndrome, the 'carcinoid syndrome' develops – the tumour produces large amounts of 5HT (not HCG), which is excreted in the urine. Pulmonary and cardiac effects are well documented.

6.25. Primary carcinoma of the bowel:

A. Occurs as frequently in the ileum as in the colon
B. The liver is a frequent site for metastases
C. Ulcerative colitis is a predisposing condition
D. The histological structure is usually a transitional cell carcinoma
E. Its metastases retain the histological features of the primary tumour

6.26. Phaeochromocytoma:

A. Arises from cells of the adrenal cortex
B. Induces glycosuria
C. Induces hypertension
D. Is an encapsulated tumour
E. Has a high content of catecholamines

6.27. The following tumours characteristically arise in the ovary:

A. Granulosa cell tumour
B. Phaeochromocytoma
C. Teratoma
D. Arrhenoblastoma
E. Disgerminoma

Answers overleaf

6.25. B, C, E.

Carcinoma of the large bowel is commoner than the small bowel. The histological features of carcinoma of the bowel are that of an adenocarcinoma.

6.26. B, C, D, E.

Phaeochromocytoma arise from cells of the adrenal medulla.

6.27. A, C, D, E.

Phaeochromochytoma is a tumour of the adrenal medulla and secretes noradrenaline and adrenaline.

6.28. Which of the following tumours are teratomata:

A. Rhabdomyoma of soft tissues
B. Mixed parotid tumour
C. 'Dermoid' cyst of the ovary
D. Nephroblastoma (Wilms' tumour)
E. Choriocarcinoma of the testis

6.29 Tumours of germ cell origin include:

A. Benign cystic teratoma
B. Granulosa cell tumour
C. Non-gestational choriocarcinoma
D. Krukenberg tumour
E. Seminoma

Answers overleaf

6.28. C, E.

The vast majority of teratoma occur in the gonads, the ovary being much more affected than the testis.

The rhabdomyoma is a tumour of connective tissue (striated muscle).

The mixed parotid tumour tends to behave for the most part like adenomata. There are all degrees of transition from adenoma to frank carcinoma in this type of neoplasm. The nephroblastoma is a tumour of the renal blastoma.

6.29. A, C, E.

Krukenberg tumours are secondary tumours of a primary mucoid carcinoma usually in the stomach or colon, but occasionally in the breast. Granulosa cell tumours are mesenchymomas and develop from the tissues of the fully formed ovary.

6.30. Hydatidiform mole is associated with increased urinary output of:

- **A.** Oestrogens
- **B.** Human chorionic gonadotrophin
- **C.** Creatinine
- **D.** Pregnanediol
- **E.** Human placental lactogen

6.31. The cause of jaundice developing in a neonate within six hours of birth may be:

- **A.** Physiological
- **B.** Atresia of the bile ducts
- **C.** Rhesus haemolytic disease
- **D.** Premature birth
- **E.** Meconium ileus

6.32. Megaloblastic anaemia may be due to:

- **A.** Deficiency of folic acid
- **B.** Hyperplasia of bone marrow
- **C.** Increased metabolic requirement
- **D.** Low serum iron
- **E.** Liver damage

Answers overleaf

6.30. A, B, D, E.

Creatinine is not produced by the trophoblastic tissue and therefore with increased activity of trophoblast there is no direct reason for an increased urinary output.

6.31. C.

Although all conditions given are associated with jaundice in the newborn the short time interval given in the opening statement excludes all except C.

6.32. A, B, C.

Any anaemia will affect the serum iron but will not be an aetiological factor. Liver damage does not cause a megaloblastic anaemia.

7. BIOCHEMISTRY

7.1. Nitrogen balance is:

A. Positive during normal pregnancy
B. Positive during prolonged immobilization
C. Negative during protein starvation
D. Negative in the untreated diabetic
E. Positive during recovery from debilitating illness

7.2. Uric acid:

A. Is the end product of purine metabolism
B. Is excreted in the bile
C. Excretion in urine is reduced by the administration of low doses of salicylates
D. Excretion in urine is enhanced by the administration of therapeutic doses of probenecid
E. Excretion in urine is reduced by the administration of corticosteroid therapy

7.3. Thiamine:

A. Is water soluble
B. Requirements are related to carbohydrate intake
C. Deficiency leads to impaired collagen formation
D. Is widely distributed in natural foods
E. Its major precursor is carotene

Answers overleaf

7.1. A, C, D, E.

Nitrogen balance is negative during prolonged immobilization.

7.2. A, B, C, D.

Uric acid is predominantly excreted in the urine but some is also excreted in the bile. Certain uricosuric drugs block reabsorption of the uric acid in the renal tubules so the amount excreted in the urine will be greater than normal. These drugs include salicylates.

7.3. A, B, D.

Severe deficiency causes the disease known as beri-beri which affects the cardio-vascular system and peripheral nerves. Carotene is not its major precursor. It occurs in yeast, wheat germ, wholemeal, wheat or rye bread, soya beans and pork fat.

7.4. Riboflavin:

A. Is water soluble
B. Is an essential dietary factor for man
C. Is widely distributed in natural foods
D. Deficiency causes defective colour vision
E. Is readily destroyed by untraviolet light

7.5. Folic acid:

A. Is fat soluble
B. Requires gastric intrinsic factor for its absorption
C. Deficiency leads to megaloblastic anaemia
D. The daily requirement for women is about 5 micrograms
E. Is in higher concentration in fetal blood than in maternal blood

7.6. Vitamin B_{12}:

A. Is fat soluble
B. Requires gastric intrinsic factor for its absorption
C. Deficiency leads to microcytic anaemia
D. The unbound fraction is excreted in the urine
E. The major dietary source is fresh vegetables

Answers overleaf

7.4. A, B, C.

Riboflavin (vitamin B_2) deficiency or excess has no effect on colour vision.

7.5. C, E.

Folic acid is water soluble and does not require the gastric intrinsic factor for its absorption. The daily requirement for women is about 40 micrograms per day, i.e. about 8–10 times the dose given in the question.

7.6. B, D.

B_{12} is water soluble and deficiency leads to a macrocytic anaemia. Foods of animal source are the only important dietary source of B_{12} e.g. milk, liver or kidney.

7.7. Ascorbic acid:

A. Is found only in foods of animal origin
B. Is water soluble
C. There are normally large stores in the pancreas
D. Is stable at high temperature
E. Is necessary for the integrity of supporting tissues

7.8. Vitamin D:

A. Is fat soluble
B. Dietary excess is excreted in the urine
C. Its major dietary source is fresh meat
D. Acts by facilitating calcium absorption from the gut
E. Deficiency leads to rickets

7.9. Vitamin E:

A. Is water soluble
B. Is a mixture of tocopherols
C. Is present in most foods
D. Is not associated with a characteristic human deficiency state
E. Excess causes infertility

Answers overleaf

7.7. B, E.

The best food sources of vitamin C are citrus fruits. The adrenal gland contains large quantities of vitamin C. Vitamin C is rapidly destroyed by heating.

7.8. A, D, E.

Ingestion of large amounts of Vitamin D have been shown to cause toxic reactions and widespread calcification of the soft tissues including lungs and kidneys. The only rich source of the vitamin is the liver and viscera of fish and the liver of animals which feed on fish.

7.9. B, C, D.

Vitamin E is fat soluble. Deficiency has been shown in animals and males to impair fertility.

7.10. The protein-bound iodine level is increased:

A. In pregnancy
B. In women taking corticosteroids
C. In hyperthyroidism
D. With increasing age
E. After absorption of large amounts of iodine

7.11. Iron utilisation in normal pregnancy:

A. During the course of a forty week gestation the fetus and placenta accumulate 400 to 500 mg of iron
B. The maternal dietary intake of elemental iron during pregnancy should be a 3–5 mg per day
C. A maximum of 10% of the dietary iron is absorbed
D. Iron is absorbed in the ferrous form
E. The administration of alkalis by mouth aids iron absorption

7.12. Under aerobic conditions, the tricarboxylic acid cycle (Krebs cycle) is an important source of:

A. Fatty acids
B. Nucleic acids
C. Adenosine triphosphate
D. Glycogen
E. Pyruvic acid

Answers overleaf

7.10. C, D, E.

The reverse occurs in B and D.

7.11. A, D.

The WHO recommend the following iron supplements for the prevention of anaemia in pregnancy.

30–60 mgm daily for populations with normal stores and supplements of iron. 120–240 mgm daily for populations without iron stores. The maximum absorption of 10% is the figure for the normal non-pregnant women, it is increased in pregnancy especially in the third trimester. Alkalies reduce absorption whilst the organic acids of food enhance absorption.

7.12. C.

The Krebs cycle results in the synthesis of adenosine triphosphate. The other substances or some of their breakdown products are involved in the cycle.

7.13. Carbohydrate metabolism in pregnancy:

A. The fasting blood glucose levels are greater than in the non-pregnant state
B. The administration of insulin to the diabetic mother suppresses fetal insulin production
C. There is an exaggerated insulin response to glucose intake
D. High levels of pituitary growth hormone reduce glucose tolerance
E. For a given injected dose of insulin the fall of blood sugar is less in the pregnant than the non-pregnant woman

7.14. In relation to carbohydrate metabolism:

A. There is an increased rate of absorption of glucose in pregnancy
B. During mid and late pregnancy there is a progressive rise in plasma insulin levels
C. The production of lactate from glucose or glycogen is dependent upon the presence of oxygen
D. Muscle glycogen is the main source of blood glucose
E. The maternal blood glucose level tends to rise during labour

7.15. Nitrogen metabolism in the healthy individual:

A. The daily obligatory nitrogen loss of an adult is less than 30 milligrams per kg body weight
B. The nitrogen content of the diet makes little or no difference to the faecal loss
C. Most of the additional nitrogen requirement in pregnancy is in the first half of pregnancy
D. A negative nitrogen balance is present when the urine is nitrogen free
E. Fibrinogen is replaced at the rate of 30–40% per day

Answers overleaf

7.13. B, C, E.

The fasting blood glucose is not greater in pregnancy. High levels of pituitary growth hormone alter glucose tolerance and may produce diabetes in the non-pregnant state.

7.14. B, E.

Although various factors increase or decrease the rate of absorption of glucose in pregnancy by itself, pregnancy is not one which increases absorption. Lactate can be produced quite independently of oxygen from glucose or glycogen. At normal glucose levels, the liver is the main producer of glucose not extra-hepatic sources.

7.15. B, E.

For the average 70 Kg man 30 mgms per Kg body weight would mean the elimination of less than 2.1 gms per day. In fact on a normal diet it would average between 10–14 gms and even on a low protein diet it would amount to 4–5 gms. The additional requirement for nitrogen is greater in the second half of pregnancy especially when one considers the protein requirements of fetal uterine growth.

Negative nitrogen balance is when loss exceeds intake. Typical examples being starvation, malnutrition, burns or trauma. It also occurs for a time following surgical operations.

8. ENDOCRINOLOGY

8.1. The following hormones are produced within the anterior lobe of the human pituitary gland:

A. Oxytocin
B. Thyroid stimulating hormone
C. Adrenocorticotrophin
D. Follicle stimulating hormone releasing hormone
E. Long acting thyroid stimulator

8.2. The hypothalamo-hypophyseal portal vascular pathway is concerned in the control of secretion by the:

A. Mammary glands
B. Posterior pituitary gland
C. Islets of Langerhans
D. Thyroid gland
E. Adrenal glands

8.3. Adrenocorticotrophic hormone:

A. Controls glucocorticoid production
B. Controls catecholamine production
C. Is increased by the secretion of a hypothalamic releasing factor
D. Is suppressed by a high level of circulating glucocorticoids
E. Shows diurnal physiological variations

Answers overleaf

8.1. B, C.

Oxytocin is produced from the posterior lobe of the pituitary gland.

FSHRH is hypothalamic in origin and LATS is an antibody developed as an auto-immune phenomena against thyroid protein. It is not produced in the anterior pituitary gland although its precise origin is unknown.

8.2. A, D, E.

By control of the secretion of trophic hormones from the anterior pituitary glands A, D and E are true answers. The pathway is not involved in insulin secretion from the islets of Langerhans which give a basal secretion of insulin. As far as the adrenal gland is concerned it is the cortex only.

8.3. A, C, D, E.

ACTH does not effect the adrenal medulla from which the catecholamines are produced.

8.4. The secretion of human growth hormone in the healthy subject is:

A. From the basophil cells of the anterior pituitary
B. Increased by hypoglycaemia
C. Increased by stress
D. Decreased by exercise in the fasting state
E. Reduced after the menopause

8.5. Pituitary follicle stimulating hormone is:

A. A glycoprotein
B. Excreted in increased amounts at the climacteric
C. Secreted by the pars intermedia of the hypophysis cerebri
D. Identical with human chorionic gonadotrophin
E. Excreted by the male

Answers overleaf

8.4. B, C.

Growth hormone comes from the eosinophil cells. It is increased by exercise *and* the fasting state. It is not reduced after the menopause and remains fairly constant.

8.5. A, B, E.

FSH is produced in the anterior lobe of the pituitary and is not identical with HCG which is predominantly luteinising in action.

8.6. Luteinising hormone:

A. Plasma levels are increased throughout pregnancy
B. Is bound to plasma proteins
C. Release is stimulated by thyrotrophin-releasing hormone
D. Plasma level is increased in post-menopausal women
E. Stimulates the synthesis of testosterone in the male

8.7. Prolactin:

A. Is secreted by the hypothalamus
B. Is necessary for mammary duct growth
C. Plasma levels are unaffected by suckling
D. Is necessary for the establishment of lactation
E. Secretion is controlled by an inhibiting factor

8.8. Antidiuretic hormone:

A. Is produced in the hypothalamus
B. Is a polypeptide
C. Is identical with oxytocin
D. Controls water reabsorption by the kidney
E. Characteristically alters renal blood flow

Answers overleaf

8.6. D, E.

Plasma levels of luteinising hormone are reduced in pregnancy because HCG from the placenta takes over. It is not bound to plasma proteins.

8.7. B, D, E.

Prolactin is found in the eosinophil cells of the anterior pituitary. Plasma levels of the hormone are affected by suckling.

8.8. A, B, D.

ADH and oxytocin are similar but not identical, the difference is in the two aminoacids. The effect on the kidney is predominantly in the renal tubules.

8.9. Endogenous vasopressin:

A. Raises blood pressure by a direct effect on the peripheral blood vessels
B. Has an antidiuretic effect
C. Causes diabetes insipidus when present in excess
D. Secretion is stimulated by morphine
E. Secretion is stimulated by alcohol

8.10. Oxytocin:

A. Has an antidiuretic effect
B. Is a steroid hormone
C. Is activated from a precursor by oxytocinase
D. Stimulates all involuntary muscle
E. Is produced by the anterior pituitary gland

8.11. Parathyroid hormone:

A. Increases the plasma phosphate level
B. Secretion is regulated by serum calcium level
C. Enhances reabsorption of calcium from bone
D. Is a polypeptide
E. Increases the urinary output of phosphate

Answers overleaf

8.9. A, B, D.

Diabetes insipidus is caused by deficiency of endogenous vasopressin. Alcohol stimulates a diuresis and therefore vasopressin production is reduced.

8.10. A.

Oxytocin is an octapeptide. Oxytocinase breaks down oxytocin. Oxytocin acts on the uterine muscle which is only one example of an involuntary muscle. It is produced in the posterior pituitary gland.

8.11. B, C, D, E.

The net effect of the renal action of an overall increase of phosphate excretion is to produce a fall in the plasma phosphate level.

8.12. Thyroxine:

A. Is essential for skeletal development
B. Stimulates oxygen consumption
C. Stimulates thyroid stimulating hormone secretion
D. Depresses cholesterol synthesis
E. Is bound to plasma proteins

8.13. Insulin inhibits:

A. Glycogen synthesis in liver
B. Glycogen deposition in skeletal muscle
C. Lipolysis
D. Protein synthesis by muscle
E. Synthesis of ribonucleic acid (RNA) in the nucleus

Answers overleaf

8.12. A, B, E.

Tyroxine inhibits TSH and stimulates cholesterol synthesis and the hepatic mechanisms that remove cholesterol from the circulation.

8.13. C.

Insulin enhances the storage of glycogen in the liver and muscle cells. A primary effect of insulin in muscle is to facilitate the transport of various substances including amino-acids into muscle in the absence of glucose and protein synthesis. The effect of insulin is to stimulate RNA synthesis in the nucleus.

8.14. Growth hormone and insulin have opposing actions on:

A. Carbohydrate uptake by muscle
B. Catabolism of fat
C. Synthesis of fat
D. Synthesis of protein
E. Somatic growth

8.15. Aldosterone:

A. Promotes the retention of sodium by the kidney
B. Promotes the excretion of potassium by the kidney
C. Potentiates the pressor effect of noradrenaline
D. Is produced by the placenta
E. Excretion is increased in proportion to circulating progesterone

Answers overleaf

8.14. A, B, C.

Both act similarly with regard to synthesis of protein and somatic growth.

8.15. A, B, C, E.

Aldosterone is only produced in the adrenal gland.

8.16. Glucocorticoids:

A. Increase protein catabolism
B. Increase the development of lymphoid tissues
C. Increase total body water
D. Reduce the secretion of adrenocorticotrophic hormone
E. Depress the blood glucose level

8.17. Aldosterone is produced by the adrenal cortex in response to:

A. Ingestion of sodium chloride
B. An increase in blood volume
C. Failure of the 'sodium pump'
D. Formation of angiotensin 11
E. Trauma

8.18. Endogenous cortisol:

A. Promotes hypoglycaemia
B. Increases the deposition of glycogen in the liver
C. Increase the uptake of amino-acids by the liver
D. Decreases nitrogen excretion
E. Promotes lipolysis

Answers overleaf

8.16. A, C, D.

Whilst glucocorticoids have an anti-inflammatory effect and prevent histamine release they do not increase the development of lymphoid tissues.

The glucocorticoids elevate the blood glucose level.

8.17. D, E.

Unlike the other corticosteroids the production of aldosterone by the adrenal is relatively uninfluenced by ACTH. In normal subjects, aldosterone is markedly increased by sodium lack, conversely the administration of sodium decreases aldosterone production. Aldosterone secretion is mainly controlled by changes in the extracellular fluid volume and independent of total body sodium, of sodium concentration, or of the sodium pump which is the mechanism responsible for the flow of sodium out of a cell and potassium into the cell. Angiostensin II is the effective substance of renin activity and this can be produced in response to conditions which cause a reduction in renal blood flow such as a fall in blood volume. Trauma exerts its effects via the hypothalamus.

8.18. B, C, E.

Cortisol elevates blood sugar (antagonistic to the effects of insulin). It exerts a protein anti-anabolic effect from gluco-neogenesis and in the presence of excess endogenous cortisol there would be a negative nitrogen balance.

8.19. Testosterone:

A. Is a steroid hormone
B. In women is largely derived from conversion of androstenedione
C. Contributes the major part of the urinary 17-oxosteroids (ketosteroids) in women
D. Inhibits follicular maturation
E. Has to undergo conversion to dihydrotestosterone before it exhibits androgenic activity

8.20. Chorionic gonadotrophin:

A. Is produced by the decidua
B. Is excreted in the urine in increasing quantities during the second trimester of normal pregnancy
C. Is a glycoprotein
D. May be measured by radioimmunoassay methods
E. May provoke cyst formation in the ovary

Answers overleaf

8.19. A, B, D, E.

In the normal healthy female 17-oxosteroids are produced entirely by the adrenal cortex. In the male by the adrenal cortex and testes. Even in males about two thirds of the 17-oxosteroids are of adrenal origin.

8.20. C, D, E.

HCG is probably produced exclusively by the Langerhans cells of the cytotrophoblast. It is likely that the syncytiotrophoblast stores the HCG produced in the deeper Langerhans layers. The peak of HCG production is about the sixtieth day of pregnancy followed by a rapid fall to a plateau which is maintained during the second trimester and there is a small secondary peak at about 30–36 weeks.

8.21. Human placental lactogen:

A. Has plasma levels in the third trimester of pregnancy which are proportional to fetal weight
B. Is present in the largest amounts in cytotrophoblast
C. Shows an increase in plasma levels when fetoplacental function is impaired
D. Is a small protein hormone (molecular weight 20,000)
E. Is responsible for the production of colostrum

8.22. Progesterone is:

A. Synthesised by trophoblast
B. Synthesised by the adrenal gland
C. Mostly excreted as pregnanetriol
D. Bound to a carrier protein in the blood
E. Synthesised from cholesterol

Answers overleaf

8.21. A, D.

HPL is present in the largest amounts in the syncytiotrophoblast though like HCG it is probably produced in the cytotrophoblast and stored in the syncytiotrophoblast. It is generally accepted that the plasma levels fall when fetoplacental function is chronically impaired. The lactogenic and somatotrophic properties of HPL from which it is named is derived from animal studies. It is reasonable to assume it plays some part in promoting human mammary gland development during pregnancy, but not the production of colostrum.

8.22. A, B, D, E.

The chief excreting product of progesterone is pregnanediol. Pregnanetriol is a metabolite of adrenocortical hormones.

9. PHYSIOLOGICAL CHANGES IN PREGNANCY AND LABOUR, OVULATION, REPRODUCTIVE AND FETAL PHYSIOLOGY

9.1. Steroid production in normal pregnancy:

A. The urinary excretion of oestriol at term is approximately eight times the value at ovulation
B. There is a thousandfold increase in the level of urinary excretion of pregnanediol between the luteal phase of the menstrual cycle and pregnancy at term
C. The cytotrophoblast is the likely site of production of placental steroids
D. The placenta is dependent upon fetal precursors for the production of progesterone
E. Urinary oestrogens form the basis for routine immunological pregnancy tests

9.2. The maternal adrenal gland in pregnancy:

A. The zona fasciculata manufactures aldosterone
B. There is a significant rise in plasma 'free cortisol' during pregnancy
C. Maximum production of cortisol occurs during the third trimester
D. The augmented cortisol production contributes to the alteration in glucose tolerance in latent diabetes
E. Administration of corticosteroids to the mother during late pregnancy may suppress the fetal adrenals causing adrenal failure in the infant after birth

Answers overleaf

9.1. C.

The excretion of oestriol at term is approximately a thousand-fold the value at the time of ovulation, whereas the pregnanediol difference is only about 8–16 fold. The placenta can produce progesterone from maternal precursors as well as fetal precursors. It is produced in conditions where no fetus is present. Immunological pregnancy tests are dependent upon the presence of HCG.

9.2. B, C, D, E.

All three cortical layers of the adrenal cortex are capable of secreting glucocorticoids and sex hormones but only the zona glomerulsa contains the enzymatic mechanism for aldosterone biosynthesis. Item B might cause confusion and depends on ones interpretation of significant rise and during pregnancy. The plasma corticosteroid levels are raised in pregnancy and occurs early in pregnancy. The protein, transcortin, that binds cortisol in plasma increases in concentration and in binding activity in pregnancy. The increased binding of cortisol therefore delays the disappearance of cortisol from the circulation and may influence its metabolism. Nevertheless in pregnancy (compared to women receiving oestrogen therapy) free cortisol does rise. The author would therefore argue that it is reasonable to accept as a true answer. The purist might say it is not significant or since it occurs early the rise thereafter is not significant – in doubt the candidate would be advised to omit an answer if penalties are given for incorrect answers. It has been left in deliberately to make this examination point, rather than for the factual knowledge.

9.3. Blood volume and blood composition in normal pregnancy:

A. The total red cell mass falls by about 20% from the normal non-pregnant value
B. The packed cell volume falls.
C. There is a rise in the iron-binding capacity
D. The blood cholesterol rises
E. The protein bound iodine level falls

9.4. Circulatory changes in a healthy woman during a normal pregnancy include:

A. A rise in cardiac output only during the second and third trimesters
B. A maximum increase in resting cardiac output of between 30 and 60%
C. A regular increase in stroke volume
D. The peripheral blood flow is reduced
E. A uterine blood flow at term of the order of 500 mls/minute

9.5. Cardiac output during normal pregnancy:

A. Is greater from the left ventricle than from the right
B. Varies with physiological changes in heart rate
C. Is reflexly reduced in a hot environment
D. Increases in the first trimester
E. Varies with stroke volume when the heart rate is constant

Answers overleaf

9.3. B, C, D.

In pregnancy, both plasma volume and the total red cell mass increase but not in the same proportion as the ratio falls. The protein bound iodine level of PBI is no more significant of thyroid activity than the high level of cholesterol is significant of low thyroid activity. The principal reason for the changes being the alteration in the proteins involved in the binding process.

9.4. B, E.

There is strong evidence that for the normal pregnant woman at rest, but not supine, that cardiac output rises during the first ten weeks of pregnancy by about 1.5 litre per minute, this rise being maintained throughout the pregnancy until term. Since there is good evidence for a rise in cardiac output of about one third accompanied by an increase in the pulse rate of about a fifth, there must be a small rise in stroke volume. Direct evidence is not available and all studies to date show wide fluctuations. There is not a regular increase in stroke volume since normal pregnancy has been recorded in women with artificial cardiac pacemakers which give a fixed heart rate. All the evidence would suggest that peripheral blood flow is increased especially in the hand and foot.

9.5. B, D, E.

The cardiac output from both ventricles would be equal as in the non-pregnant state. In general there is no increase with moderate changes in temperature but an increase would be expected as in the non-pregnant woman in a very hot environment.

9.6. Haemopoiesis in pregnancy:

A. Throughout pregnancy there is a parallel increase in maternal plasma volume and red cell mass
B. If diet is adequate the total maternal red cell volume has increased by about 250 ml in late pregnancy
C. The fetus and placenta require about 0.5 gram of elemental iron during the course of pregnancy
D. 300 micrograms folic acid daily is an adequate dietary supplement for normal pregnancy
E. The average maximum increase in plasma volume during pregnancy is about 500 ml

9.7. In late pregnancy an increase occurs in the blood concentration of:

A. Fibrinogen
B. Albumin
C. Sodium
D. Transferrin
E. Cholesterol

Answers overleaf

9.6. B, C, D.

There is a marked discrepancy in the relative increase in maternal plasma volume and red cell mass. The plasma volume increases on average by at least 1250 ml above the non-pregnant level of 2600 ml

9.7. A, D, E.

Concentration reflects the total amount of a substance within a given volume. Whilst both the blood volume and the actual amount of a given substance may be increased in late pregnancy it to some extent depends on the relative quantities of each. Fibrinogen increases in pregnancy by 1–2 grammes per litre and the total amount of fibrinogen increases from about 10 grammes in the non-pregnant woman to 28 grammes in the late pregnancy. Albumin falls throughout pregnancy and the overall fall is of the order of 10 grammes per litre. In normal pregnancy there is a small but consistent fall in the concentration of most serum electrolytes including sodium.

9.8. Which of the following changes occur in the mother during normal pregnancy?

A. Renal blood flow increases only during the last trimester
B. There is an increase in aldosterone secretion
C. The blood urea level falls below 25 milligrams per 100 ml
D. The concentration of sodium in body fluids is above that of non-pregnant women
E. Respiratory tidal volume falls

9.9. The immediate effects of coitus in the human female normally include:

A. Change of the vaginal pH to a level above 6.5
B. Ejaculation from the clitoris
C. A pressure gradient between the vagina and uterine cavity
D. Secretion of 5-hydroxytryptamine from the cells of the vaginal epithelium
E. Elevation of blood pressure

Answers overleaf

9.8. B, C.

Renal plasma and blood flow increase significantly early in pregnancy.
In pregnancy, there is a small but consistent fall in sodium concentration.
The respiratory total volume increases.

9.9. A, C, E.

There is no ejaculation from the clitoris. It contains erectile tissue and is the homologue of the dorsal part of the penis. There is no evidence for the secretion of 5-hydroxytryptamine from the cells of vaginal epithelium although there is a copious transudate in the vagina.

9.10. Ovulation in the human:

A. Is associated with a surge of luteinising hormone
B. Is characteristically followed by the development of secretory endometrium
C. Is associated with an increase in motility of the Fallopian tubes
D. Is associated with a sustained fall in basal body temperature
E. Is followed by a rise in urinary pregnanetriol

9.11. The following findings on the twenty-third day of a normal twenty-eight day menstrual cycle provide strong evidence that ovulation has occurred:

A. Cervical mucus with positive arborization when dried on a glass slide
B. Subnuclear vacuolation apparent on endometrium biopsy
C. High cornification index in vaginal cytology preparations
D. High level of total oestrogens in a twenty-four hour specimen of urine
E. Presence of an apparently healthy corpus luteum in an ovary

9.12. In a normal human menstrual cycle the corpus luteum:

A. Remains active for 3–4 weeks
B. Is maintained by human chorionic gonadotrophin
C. Secretes progesterone
D. Secretes pregnanediol
E. Secretes oestrogen

Answers overleaf

9.10. A, B, C.

There may be a small fall followed by a rise in temperature but the fall is not sustained. Pregnanetriol is a metabolite of adrenocortical hormones and therefore not related to ovulation.

9.11. B, E.

A positive arborization test will be negative at this time in a twenty-eight day menstrual cycle. The cornification index will be low and the levels of total oestrogens would have fallen from the peak levels at the time of ovulation.

9.12. C, E.

In the absence of pregnancy the corpus luteum only remains active for about ten days then degenerates. It is not maintained by HCG. Pregnanediol is a breakdown production of progesterone and is usually measured in the urine. Not all pregnanediol is derived from progesterone, there are other precursors in the body.

9.13. The main fetal contributions to oestriol production are:

A. Dehydroepiandrosterone sulphate
B. 16α -hydroxy-dehydroepiandrosterone
C. Oestrone
D. Oestradiol – 17β
E. Oestriol-17-glucosiduronate

9.14. An excess of amniotic fluid is associated with:

A. Fetal meningocele
B. Maternal diabetes insipidus
C. Fetal renal agenesis
D. Fetal duodenal atresia
E. An anencephalic fetus

9.15. Lowering of the pH of a fetal scalp blood sample occurs:

A. When the second stage of labour is prolonged
B. With prolonged exposure of the sample to room air before measurement
C. When the sample is taken from an area with a large caput succedaneum
D. In maternal acidosis
E. When there is excess heparin in the collecting tube

Answers overleaf

9.13. A, B.

In light of present accepted knowledge the two correct answers indicate the main fetal contribution. It is accepted that about nine tenths of the precursors of placental oestriol are produced in the fetal adrenals.

9.14. A, D, E.

There is no increase in amniotic fluid in maternal diabetes insipidus and there is a marked reduction in fetal renal agenesis. In the later condition there is also usually an associated abnormality of the amniotic membrane.

9.15. A, C, D, E.

The pH in general should be measured as soon as possible and with increased oxygenation of venous scalp blood the pH would tend to be elevated not lowered.

9.16. In the human uterus:

A. Activity increases in amplitude during the secretory phase of the menstrual cycle
B. Spontaneous activity is absent during the first and second trimesters of pregnancy
C. Denervation results in a reduction of muscle contractility
D. The response of the non-pregnant uterus to oxytocin is poor
E. Noradrenaline increases the contractility of the pregnant uterus

9.17. In normal labour:

A. Endogenous oxytocin is responsible for the initiation of uterine contractions
B. There is a progressive increase in plasma cortisol
C. The uterine contractions cause no rise in intra -uterine hydrostatic pressure
D. The amplitude of uterine contractions is increased by turning the mother from her back to lying on her side
E. During the first stage of labour the maternal arterial pressure rises during each uterine contraction

Answers overleaf

9.16. D, E.

Uterine activity as far as present evidence goes suggests activity is augmented during sexual stimulation, menstruation and during pregnancy. The secretory activity appears to be less during the secretory phase of the menstrual cycle. Experimental evidence of various types of muscle tissue including the uterus shows that denervation by itself does not result in a reduction of muscle contractility.

9.17. B, D, E.

A sudden change in endogenous oxytocin has not as yet been proven as the cause for the abrupt change from spontaneous Braxton-Hicks contractions to the contractions of labour with cervical dilatation. Many factors have been and are being studied including the fetal endocrine system, uterine volume, oxytocin concentration, myometrial sensitivity to mention a few. Any reasonable monitoring device nowadays used in labour will show alteration and rise in intrauterine pressure.

10. PHYSIOLOGY

10.1. Which of the following buffers are found in both the plasma and erythrocytes:

A. Albumin
B. Bicarbonate
C. Globulin
D. Inorganic phosphate
E. Organic phosphate

10.2. Which of the following statements concerning the plasma hydrogen ion concentration (pH) are true or false:

A. An increase in the partial pressure of carbon dioxide tends to reduce pH
B. The protein-buffer system is the most important in the extra-cellular fluid
C. pH 7.4 corresponds to a mean (H+) of 40 mEq/litre
D. A change in the concentration of bicarbonate ion moves the pH in the opposite direction
E. The ratio (HCO_3/H_2CO_3) has to be kept at approximately 40/1 to maintain a pH of 7.4

10.3. The pH of blood:

A. In the carotid artery is normally less than that of cerebrospinal fluid
B. Rises as a result of profuse diarrhoea
C. Rises with repeated vomiting of gastric contents
D. In the right atrium is lower than in the left atrium
E. Is lower in the renal vein than in the renal artery

Answers overleaf

10.1. B, D.

The answers are self explanatory.

10.2. A.

The principal buffers in the extracellular fluid are haemoglobin, protein and bicarbonate. Haemoglobin has six times the buffering capacity of the plasma proteins. The normal hydrogen ion concentration (H^+) in plasma is 0.00004 mEq/litre. The pH, i.e. the negative logarithm of 0.00004 is 7.4. For each pH of 0.1 less than 7.0 the (H^+) is increased tenfold and for each pH above it is decreased tenfold. In extreme acidosis the (H^+) is 0.0001 which corresponds to a pH of 7.0.

In item D the reverse applies, the move is in the same direction. The rate of HCO_3/H_2CO_3 is about 20/1 to maintain a pH of 7.4.

10.3. C, D.

The pH in the carotid artery is normally higher than in CSF. Profuse diarrhoea would result in acidosis and therefore the pH would fall. The pH in the renal vein is higher than in the renal artery.

10.4. In muscle capillary circulation:

A. Blood pH rises
B. Bicarbonate ions pass from the red cells to the plasma
C. The concentration of chloride ions in the red cells falls
D. The saturation of haemoglobin with oxygen varies inversely with blood pH
E. The blood nitrogen content remains unchanged

10.5. Sodium:

A. In conditions of sodium depletion there is a decrease in aldosterone secretion
B. The daily intake of sodium in the diet in temperate climates is 5–20 grammes
C. Sodium balance is finely adjusted by the proximal tubule of the kidney
D. There is an obligatory loss of sodium in the urine
E. Is the principal cation of the intracellular fluid

10.6. The following conditions cause metabolic acidosis:

A. Prolonged vomiting
B. Chronic renal failure
C. Hyperventilation
D. Uretero-colic anastomosis
E. Respiratory distress syndrome of the newborn

Answers overleaf

10.4. B, E.

The blood pH falls and the concentration of chloride ions in the RBC's increases. The saturation of haemoglobin with oxygen varies directly with the blood pH.

10.5. B, D.

Aldosterone secretion is increased in sodium depletion. Variations in sodium excretion are affected by changes in the amount filtered, by the amount re-absorbed in the renal tubules or both mechanisms.

Potassium is the principle cation of the intracellular fluid.

10.6. B, D, E.

Metabolic alkalosis is more likely to occur after prolonged vomiting. Respiratory alkalosis occurs with hyperventilation.

10.7. In a normal non-pregnant human adult female the extra-cellular fluid:

A. Has a total volume of 12–13 litres
B. Forms a greater proportion of total body weight in the obese than in the lean subject
C. Has a sodium content similar to blood plasma
D. Is isotonic with sea water
E. Volume is regulated primarily by the kidneys

10.8. Functions of lymph include:

A. The return of protein to the circulation
B. Generation of lymphocytes
C. The regulation of the interstitial fluid pressure
D. The return of excess tissue fluid to the blood
E. Generation of antibodies

10.9. In the normal cardiac cycle:

A. The peak pressure in the pulmonary arterial system is approximately one-twentieth of that in the systemic arterial system
B. The first heart sound is caused by closure of the mitral and aortic valves
C. Atrial contraction occurs in the early part of ventricular filling
D. The stroke volume at rest is 60–100 mls
E. Sympathetic stimulation increases the heart rate

Answers overleaf

10.7. A, C, E.

In B the reverse is true. Extra cellular fluid is not isotonic with sea water which contains much more salt.

10.8. A, C, D.

Lymph is tissue fluid that enters lymphatic vessels.

Lymphocytes enter the circulation principally through the lymphatics but they are not generated from lymph and neither are antibodies.

10.9. D, E.

The peak pressure difference between the pulmonary and systemic circulation is approximately a tenth. The first sound is caused by the closure of the mitral and tricuspid valves and the second sound by the aortic and pulmonary valves. Atrial contraction occurs in the late part of ventricular filling.

10.10. Systolic arterial blood pressure is:

A. Unaffected by changes in posture
B. Directly related to the level of plasma renin
C. Unaffected by the peripheral vascular resistance
D. Affected by the venous return to the heart
E. Lowered by 5-hydroxytryptamine

10.11. Active erythropoietic tissue:

A. First appears in the bone marrow during the last three months of intrauterine life
B. Occupies the whole bone marrow at birth
C. Is replaced by fat in the long bones of the healthy adult
D. Is not found in the vertebrae of adults
E. Is present in the flat bones of the healthy adult

10.12. Substances essential to the development of red blood cells are:

A. Folinic acid
B. Ascorbic acid
C. Nicotinic acid
D. Cyanocobalamin (Vitamin B_{12})
E. Desoxyribonucleic acid (DNA)

Answers overleaf

10.10. D.

Blood pressure (BP) is affected by posture and peripheral vascular resistance. It is indirectly related to the level of renin and its subsequent activity

5-hydroxytrptamine causes vasoconstriction and therefore would not be associated with a reduction in BP

10.11. B, C, E.

Active tissue is present early in intrauterine life and is present in the vertebrae of adults.

10.12. A, B, D, E.

Nicotinic acid is a component of coenzymes I and II but not essential to the development of RBC's.

10.13. Fetal haemoglobin:

A. Is not formed before sixteen weeks of gestation
B. Is more resistant than adult haemoglobin to denaturation by alkalis
C. Comprises 85–95% of the haemoglobin in the new born
D. Is found in a concentration of less than 5% in an infant of eight weeks.
E. Is found in adult patients with thalassaemia

10.14. Iron metabolism in normal adults:

A. The human body contains 10–15 grammes of iron
B. Iron is transported in the blood in the ferrous state
C. The total iron binding capacity of the plasma is between 300 and 400 micrograms per 100 ml of blood
D. The solubility of iron is decreased by phytates
E. Iron deficiency anaemia is a macrocytic anaemia

10.15. Plasmin:

A. Is responsible for the formation of a fibrin net
B. Is formed from plasminogen by tissue activators
C. Produces fibrinogen degradation products (FDP) when incubated with fibrinogen
D. Is susceptible to inhibition by an anti plasmin
E. May lyse adreno-corticotrophic hormone

Answers overleaf

10.13. B, C, E.

Fetal haemoglobin is found well before sixteen weeks gestation and normally disappears more or less completely during the first year of life.

There would be more than 5% present in an infant of eight weeks.

10.14. A, C, D.

The iron in the blood is bound to a beta globulin called transferin or siderophilin. Iron is absorbed in the ferous state. Iron deficiency anaemia is microcytic.

10.15. B, C, D, E.

Plasmin lyses the clot.

10.16. Blood coagulation may be delayed by:

A. Deficiency of prothrombin
B. Deficiency of factor IX (Christmas factor)
C. Heparin
D. Calcium citrate
E. Potassium oxalate

10.17. Blood from the following donors will be agglutinated if transfused into the recipients indicated:

	Donor	Recipient
A.	Blood group O	Blood group AB
B.	Blood group AB	Blood group O
C.	Blood group A	Blood group AB
D.	Blood group B	Blood group O
E.	Blood group A	Blood group B

Answers overleaf

10.16. A, B, C, D, E.

All true items.

10.17. B, D, E.

The answers are self-explanatory if one recalls the basic knowledge about blood groups and transfusion reactions.

10.18. In a normal man breathing quietly at rest the partial pressure of:

A. Carbon dioxide in alveolar air is 2–3 times that in the room air
B. Carbon dioxide in pulmonary arterial blood is greater than in alveolar air
C. Water vapour in alveolar air is less than half that of alveolar CO_2
D. Nitrogen in expired air is greater than in inspired air
E. Oxygen in pulmonary arterial blood is less than in alveolar air

10.19. The respiratory centre:

A. Is situated in the medulla oblongata
B. Is regulated by afferent vagal impulses
C. Ceases rhythmical activity if both vagi are cut
D. Responds to impulses from the cerebral cortex
E. Is sensitive to pH alteration in the blood

10.20. Angiotensin 11:

A. Is derived from renin
B. Is a powerful hypertensive agent
C. Is produced by the renal juxtaglomerular apparatus
D. Causes contraction of vascular smooth muscle
E. Provokes the release of vasopressin

Answers overleaf

10.18. B, E.

The partial pressure of CO_2 in the alveoli is of the order of 40 compared with about 0.3–0.4 which means the difference is at least tenfold. The water pressure is slightly greater than that of alveolar CO_2. There is more nitrogen in inspired air.

10.19. A, B, D, E.

The false answer is not true because activity will still continue albeit at a different level.

10.20. B, D.

Angiotensin 11 is derived from angiotensin 1 by a converting enzyme. Angiotensin 1 is liberated by the action of renin which is secreted from the juxta glomerular cells. It may provoke release of aldosterone from the adrenal cortex but does not provoke the release of vasopressin.

10.21. In a healthy normotensive twenty year old non-pregnant woman eating a varied diet:

- **A.** Renin production is lower when standing than when sitting or lying down
- **B.** Renin is produced by the juxta-glomerular cells in the kidney
- **C.** Renin is necessary for the production of angiotensin 1
- **D.** Angiotensin 11 has a direct action on the renal tubules
- **E.** Aldosterone secretion is increased after taking most 'combined' oral contraceptives

10.22. The concentration of urine:

- **A.** Is due to active reabsorption of water
- **B.** Is completed in the loop of Henle
- **C.** Occurs progressively along the proximal tubule
- **D.** Is dependent on antidiuretic hormone
- **E.** Is related to the osmolality of the medullary interstitial fluid

10.23. The following substances may be used to measure the glomerular filtration rate:

- **A.** Vitamin B_{12}
- **B.** Insulin
- **C.** Glucose
- **D.** Inulin
- **E.** Para-aminohippuric acid

Answers overleaf

10.21. B, C, E.

Renin secretion is higher on standing than when sitting or lying supine.

Angiotensin 11 acts directly on the aldosterone producing cells of the zona glomerulosa of the adrenal cortex.

10.22. D, E.

Water is reabsorbed secondary to the active reabsorption of solutes in the proximal tubule and therefore varies. The descending limb of the loop of Henle is permeable to water and not to solute.

The ascending limb of the loop of Henle is impermeable to water but active transfer of sodium chloride occurs. ADH acts on the distal tube and collecting tubules under normal circumstances. The urine will ultimately be hyposmotic if hypotonic urine is to be excreted and hyperosmotic if water is to be conserved and hypertonic urine is to be excreted.

10.23. A, D.

The characteristics of a substance suitable for measuring the glomerular filtration rate by determining its clearance are that it is freely filtered, not reabsorbed or secreted by the tubules, not metabolised, not stored in the kidney, not protein bound (substances bound to albumin and globulin are not filtered) non-toxic, have no effect on filtration rate, and preferably be easy to measure in plasma and urine. Inulin is the most common substance although Vitamin B_{12} would fit the above criteria. Creatinine which is used has limitations and is not precise enough for accurate determinations. Some creatinine is secreted by the tubules and some reabsorbed by the tubules.

10.24. Renal plasma flow is:

A. Between 600–800 ml per minute
B. Increased by vigorous exercise
C. Increased in normal pregnancy
D. Reduced when lying down
E. Increased in water depletion

10.25. The human milk ejection reflex:

A. Has a humoral afferent arc
B. Is mediated by oxytocin
C. Is an inborn reflex
D. Is inhibited by adrenaline
E. Effects the myo-epithelial cells of the alveoli

10.26. During the climateric:

A. Oestrogens are produced in the adrenal cortex
B. There is a decreased secretion of follicle stimulating hormone
C. There is an increased secretion of luteinizing hormone
D. The vaginal pH is increased
E. The endometrium becomes unresponsive to the action of oestrogens

Answers overleaf

10.24. A, C.

The reverse is true for B, D and E respectively.

10.25. B, D, E.

The milk ejection is not an inborn reflex and normally initiated by a neuroendocrine reflex. The receptors involved are the touch receptors which are plentiful in the breast especially around the nipple. The infant suckling the breast stimulates the touch receptors, the paraventricular nuclei are stimulated, oxytocin is released, and the milk is expressed into the sinuses ready to flow into the mouth of the infant.

10.26. A, C, D.

The greatly reduced production of oestrogen as a result of cessation of ovarian function means that its inhibiting action on gonadotrophin secretion is minimal and the gonadotrophin levels are elevated. The endometrium can be stimulated by exogenous oestrogens to produce withdrawal bleeding after the climacteric. It is to some extent dose dependent and may be above the therapeutic level of therapy given during the climacteric.

10.27. In the stomach:

A. Twenty to twenty five per cent of the products of ingested protein are absorbed
B. Production of hydrochloric acid depends on the activity of carbonic anhydrase
C. Mechanical activity increases when fat enters the duodenum
D. Mechanical activity increases in response to noradrenaline
E. There are oxyntic (parietal) cells

10.28. In fat metabolism:

A. Digestion and absorption of fat are impaired in the absence of pancreatic enzymes
B. Digestion of fat begins after contact with saliva
C. Bile salts aid the emulsification of fat
D. Lipaemia represents an abnormal state of fat absorption
E. Fat absorption occurs both into the blood stream and lymphatic system

10.29. Which of the following nerve fibres produce their characteristic physiological effect by releasing acetylcholine:

A. Preganglionic fibres of the sympathetic system
B. Postganglionic fibres of the sympathetic system
C. Preganglionic fibres of the parasympathetic system
D. Postganglionic fibres of the parasympathetic system
E. Motor fibres to skeletal muscle

Answers overleaf

10.27. B, E.

The chief digestive function of the stomach is the partial digestion of protein. Absorption is therefore negligible. In the case of items C and D, activity is decreased by the respective substances.

10.28. A, C, E.

The saliva is relatively unimportant in digestion and has no effect on fat. Small fat globules are present in the blood after meals so that the plasma has a milky appearance which is known as a lipaemia. It is not an abnormal state, it is a normal event in the absorption of fat.

10.29. A, C, D, E.

The chemical transmitter at most postganglionic sympathetic endings is noradrenaline (norepinephrine).

10.30. A nerve impulse in an axon:

- **A.** Can only travel in one direction
- **B.** Requires energy
- **C.** Is conducted along an axon at approximately the speed of light
- **D.** Is conducted at the same speed as in large axons
- **E.** Is not delayed at synapse before transmission

Answers overleaf

10.30. B.

A nerve impulse can travel in either direction. The nerve impulse is relatively slow compared with the speed of light.

In general, the greater the diameter of a given nerve fibre, the greater the speed of conduction. There is a definite time interval (albeit in absolute time short) at a synapse before transmission.

11. STATISTICS AND EPIDEMIOLOGY

11.1. In the statistical analysis of any group of numerical observations:

A. The mean is always less than the mode
B. The median value always lies at the mid-point of the range
C. The standard deviation is independent of the total number of observations
D. The variance is twice the standard deviation
E. There are the same number of observations greater than and less than the median value

11.2. In a study of 1000 live born infants the mean birth weight was 3400 grammes, with a standard deviation of 300 grammes:

A. The heaviest infant would weigh 3700 grammes
B. 95% of the weights should lie between 2800 grammes and 4000 grammes
C. No infant would weigh less than 2800 grammes
D. There would be 500 infants weighing less than 3400 grammes
E. Up to 25 infants could weigh over 4000 grammes

11.3. In a sample of 400 women of child-bearing age it was found that their heights were distributed normally about a mean of 63 inches with a standard deviation of 2.4 inches:

A. One would expect the modal height to be approximately 63 inches
B. The variance of this sample of heights is not likely to exceed 1.2 inches
C. One would expect 66% of women in the sample to have a height between 60.6 inches and 65.4 inches
D. The standard error of the mean is 0.12 inches
E. The probability that the true mean height of the population from which this sample was drawn lies between 62.76 inches and 63.24 inches is 0.95

Answers overleaf

11.1. E.

The mode is the most frequent value but it will obviously not always correspond with the arithmetic mean which in a symmetrical distribution is very close to the most frequent value. Most distributions are however not strictly symmetrical. For a group of uneven numbers the mean falls between the two higher values of the series and for an even number it is the highest value. The standard deviation is dependent on the total number of observations. The square root of the variance is known as the standard deviation. The median is the value in which 50% of the observations fall above it and 50% below it.

11.2. B, E.

In a normal distribution, 95% of the infants weigh between 2800 grammes and 4000, therefore the heaviest infant cannot weigh 3700 grammes and some infants must weigh less than 2800 grammes. It is impossible to say how many infants actually weigh 3400 grammes but it would be less than 500 even if only 499! With a normal distribution, 2.5% of infants (25) would weigh less than 2800 grammes and the same number above 4000 grammes. This type of question can be varied giving a number of individuals (or observations) and the mean value and standard deviation.

11.3. A, C, D, E.

The square root of the variance is known as the standard deviation. The standard deviation is given as 2.4 inches and it is suggested that the variance cannot exceed 1.2 inches which 1/2 of the standard deviation. The variance must be $2.4 \times 2.4 = 5.76$.

11.4. In describing the specific epidemiological characteristics of a population with a condition:

A. The total rate is the ratio $\frac{\text{all cases in the population}}{\text{total number of the population}}$
B. The prevalence is the number of new cases in a stated period of time
C. For acute diseases, the incidence and prevalence are similar
D. In chronic disease, the incidence is higher than the prevalence
E. The standardized mortality ratio is the mortality rate of a specific group expressed as a percentage of the mortality rate of the total population

11.5. The true incidence of a disease may be calculated from:

A. The number of cases in each group diagnosed in a hospital each year
B. The proportion of hospital beds occupied by patients with the disease
C. The proportion of persons with the disease in a random sample of the population
D. The number of new cases occurring each year in a defined population
E. Mortality rates if the case fatality ratio is high

Answers overleaf

11.4. A, B, C, E.

Although in many chronic diseases the disease prevalence is small compared with the total population, the incidence will not be higher than the prevalence.

The true answers to this and the next question give some basic facts regarding possible epidemiology questions.

11.5. D, E.

The true answer to item D explains why the answers to A, B and C are incorrect. The final item gives an example of a reasonable comparison of fatal cases with a defined group. This question and the previous one are presented to indicate the difficulties that occur in finding suitable questions for candidates.

ANSWER SHEETS

The answer pages are presented in a simple form and therefore different from a computer type of answer page encountered in examinations. Mark with a tick (√) those answers you think are 'true' and those which you think are 'false'. Do not mark either part if you are uncertain of the answer or do not know the answer. Award yourself one mark for each correct answer (whether marked true or false) and deduct a mark for each incorrect answer. This will enable you to obtain an idea of your knowledge of the questions in individual chapters.

A slightly more sophisticated idea of computer marking can be gained by noting the total number of questions per chapter and the total number of true answers. For example in Chapter 1 there are 38 questions with 190 individual items of factual knowledge for which answers are required. 94 items are true, 96 false.

You can work out the number of correct items (true or false) out of the 190 and express it as a percentage. Similarly you should work out the percentage of answers you have marked incorrectly and deduct it from those given correctly. This will emphasize the effect of incorrect answers on the overall result.

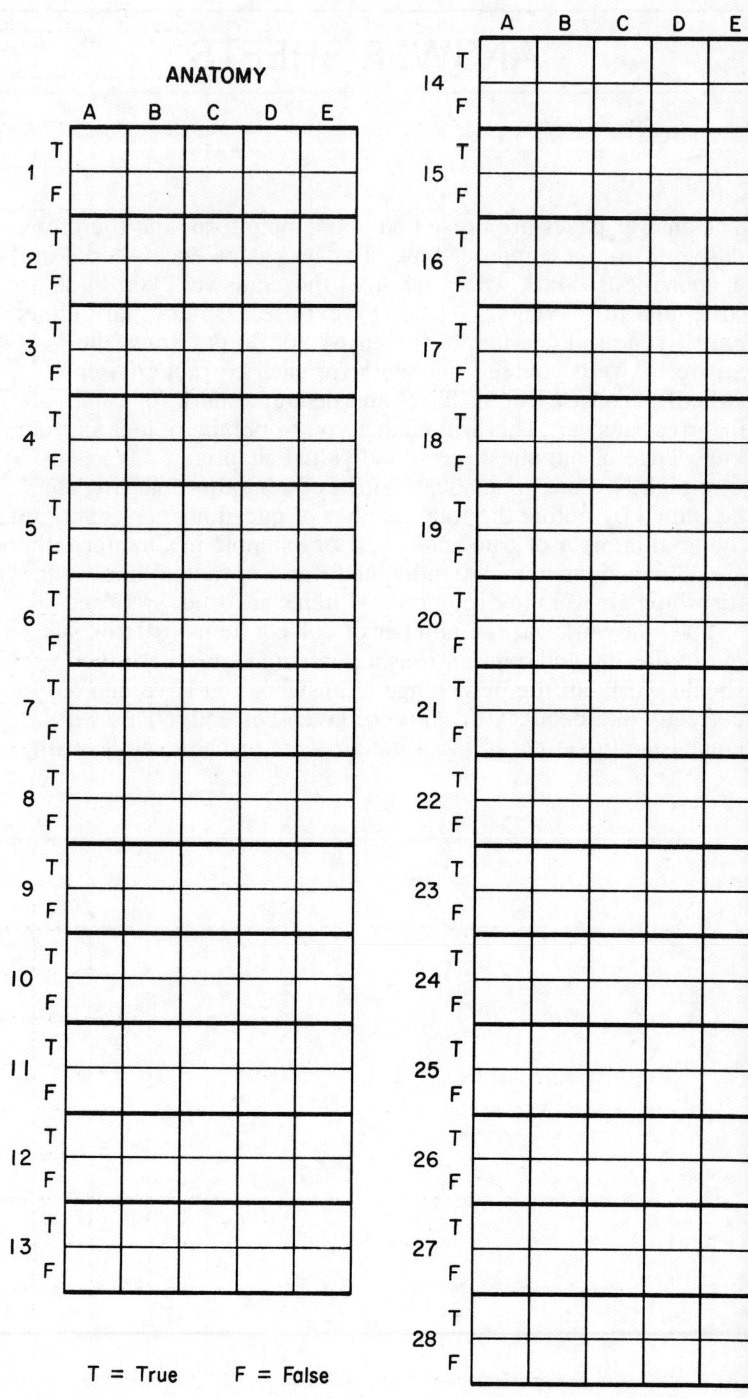

ANATOMY

		A	B	C	D	E
1	T					
	F					
2	T					
	F					
3	T					
	F					
4	T					
	F					
5	T					
	F					
6	T					
	F					
7	T					
	F					
8	T					
	F					
9	T					
	F					
10	T					
	F					
11	T					
	F					
12	T					
	F					
13	T					
	F					

		A	B	C	D	E
14	T					
	F					
15	T					
	F					
16	T					
	F					
17	T					
	F					
18	T					
	F					
19	T					
	F					
20	T					
	F					
21	T					
	F					
22	T					
	F					
23	T					
	F					
24	T					
	F					
25	T					
	F					
26	T					
	F					
27	T					
	F					
28	T					
	F					

T = True F = False

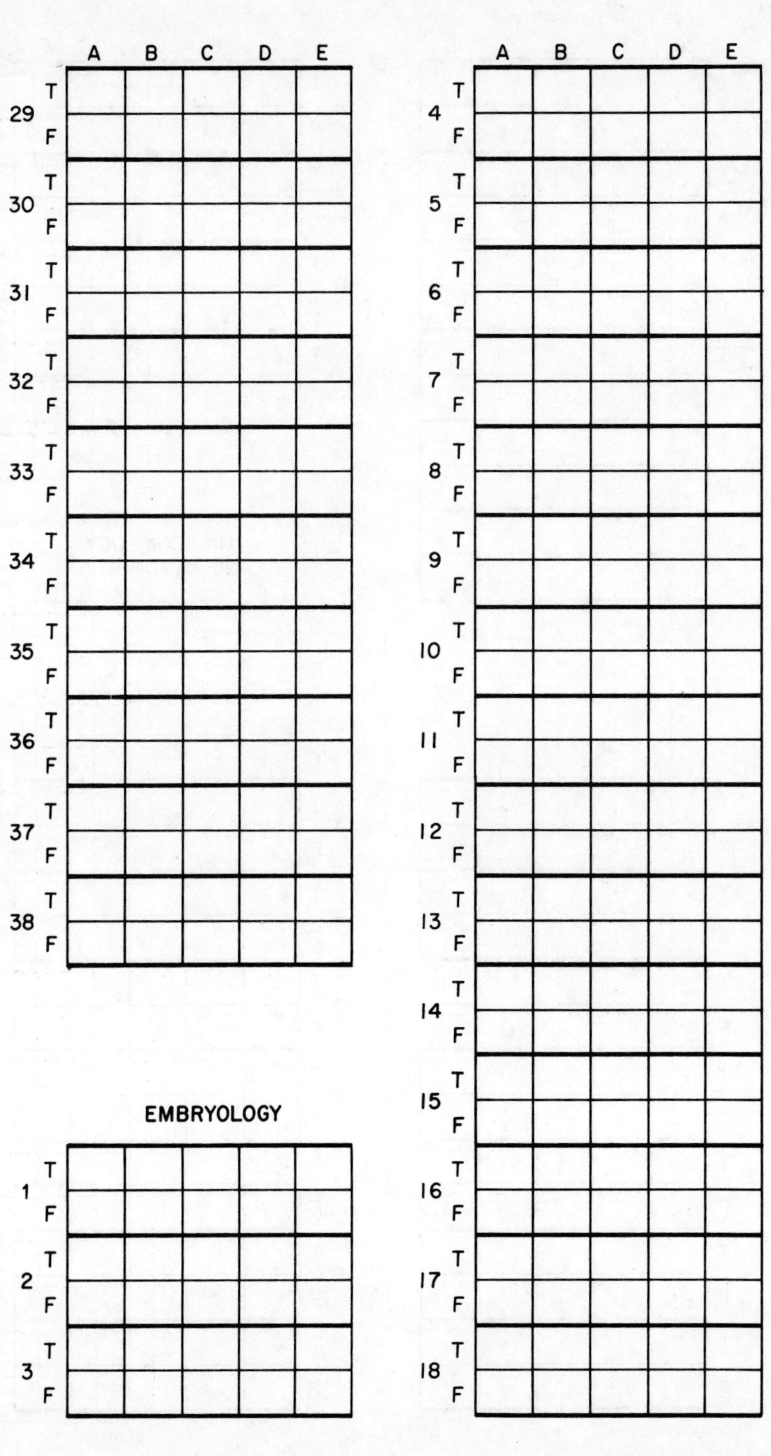
A B C D E
29 T F
30 T F
31 T F
32 T F
33 T F
34 T F
35 T F
36 T F
37 T F
38 T F
EMBRYOLOGY
1 T F
2 T F
3 T F
A B C D E
4 T F
5 T F
6 T F
7 T F
8 T F
9 T F
10 T F
11 T F
12 T F
13 T F
14 T F
15 T F
16 T F
17 T F
18 T F

		A	B	C	D	E
19	T					
	F					
20	T					
	F					
21	T					
	F					
22	T					
	F					
23	T					
	F					
24	T					
	F					

GENETICS

		A	B	C	D	E
1	T					
	F					
2	T					
	F					
3	T					
	F					
4	T					
	F					
5	T					
	F					
6	T					
	F					
7	T					
	F					

		A	B	C	D	E
8	T					
	F					
9	T					
	F					
10	T					
	F					
11	T					
	F					

MICROBIOLOGY AND IMMUNOLOGY

		A	B	C	D	E
1	T					
	F					
2	T					
	F					
3	T					
	F					
4	T					
	F					
5	T					
	F					
6	T					
	F					
7	T					
	F					
8	T					
	F					
9	T					
	F					

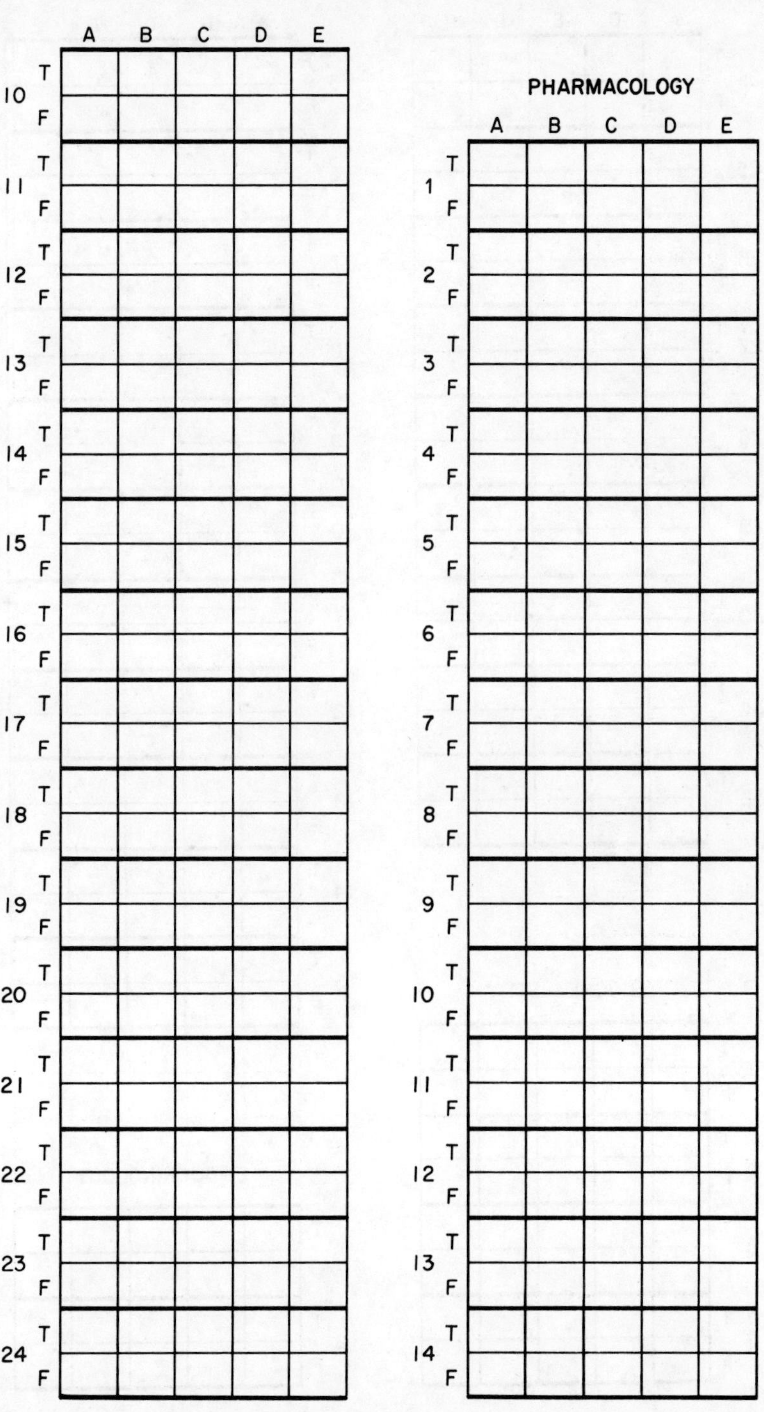

		A	B	C	D	E
10	T					
	F					
11	T					
	F					
12	T					
	F					
13	T					
	F					
14	T					
	F					
15	T					
	F					
16	T					
	F					
17	T					
	F					
18	T					
	F					
19	T					
	F					
20	T					
	F					
21	T					
	F					
22	T					
	F					
23	T					
	F					
24	T					
	F					

PHARMACOLOGY

		A	B	C	D	E
1	T					
	F					
2	T					
	F					
3	T					
	F					
4	T					
	F					
5	T					
	F					
6	T					
	F					
7	T					
	F					
8	T					
	F					
9	T					
	F					
10	T					
	F					
11	T					
	F					
12	T					
	F					
13	T					
	F					
14	T					
	F					

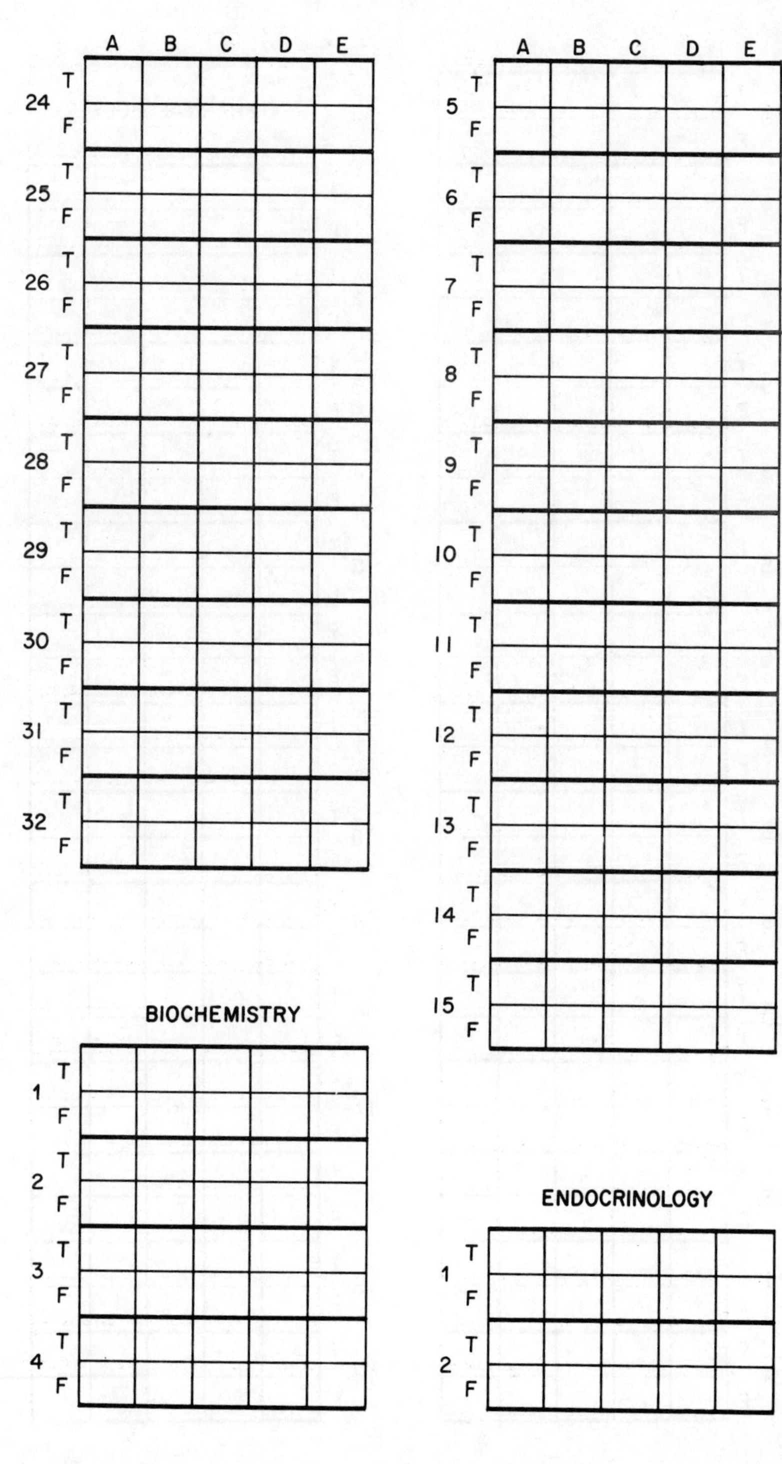

		A	B	C	D	E
24	T					
	F					
25	T					
	F					
26	T					
	F					
27	T					
	F					
28	T					
	F					
29	T					
	F					
30	T					
	F					
31	T					
	F					
32	T					
	F					

BIOCHEMISTRY

1	T					
	F					
2	T					
	F					
3	T					
	F					
4	T					
	F					

		A	B	C	D	E
5	T					
	F					
6	T					
	F					
7	T					
	F					
8	T					
	F					
9	T					
	F					
10	T					
	F					
11	T					
	F					
12	T					
	F					
13	T					
	F					
14	T					
	F					
15	T					
	F					

ENDOCRINOLOGY

1	T					
	F					
2	T					
	F					

		A	B	C	D	E
15	T					
	F					
16	T					
	F					
17	T					
	F					
18	T					
	F					
19	T					
	F					

PATHOLOGY

		A	B	C	D	E
1	T					
	F					
2	T					
	F					
3	T					
	F					
4	T					
	F					
5	T					
	F					
6	T					
	F					
7	T					
	F					
8	T					
	F					

		A	B	C	D	E
9	T					
	F					
10	T					
	F					
11	T					
	F					
12	T					
	F					
13	T					
	F					
14	T					
	F					
15	T					
	F					
16	T					
	F					
17	T					
	F					
18	T					
	F					
19	T					
	F					
20	T					
	F					
21	T					
	F					
22	T					
	F					
23	T					
	F					

		A	B	C	D	E
3	T					
	F					
4	T					
	F					
5	T					
	F					
6	T					
	F					
7	T					
	F					
8	T					
	F					
9	T					
	F					
10	T					
	F					
11	T					
	F					
12	T					
	F					
13	T					
	F					
14	T					
	F					
15	T					
	F					
16	T					
	F					
17	T					
	F					

		A	B	C	D	E
18	T					
	F					
19	T					
	F					
20	T					
	F					
21	T					
	F					
22	T					
	F					

PHYSIOLOGICAL CHANGES IN PREGNANCY. OVULATION

1	T					
	F					
2	T					
	F					
3	T					
	F					
4	T					
	F					
5	T					
	F					
6	T					
	F					
7	T					
	F					
8	T					
	F					

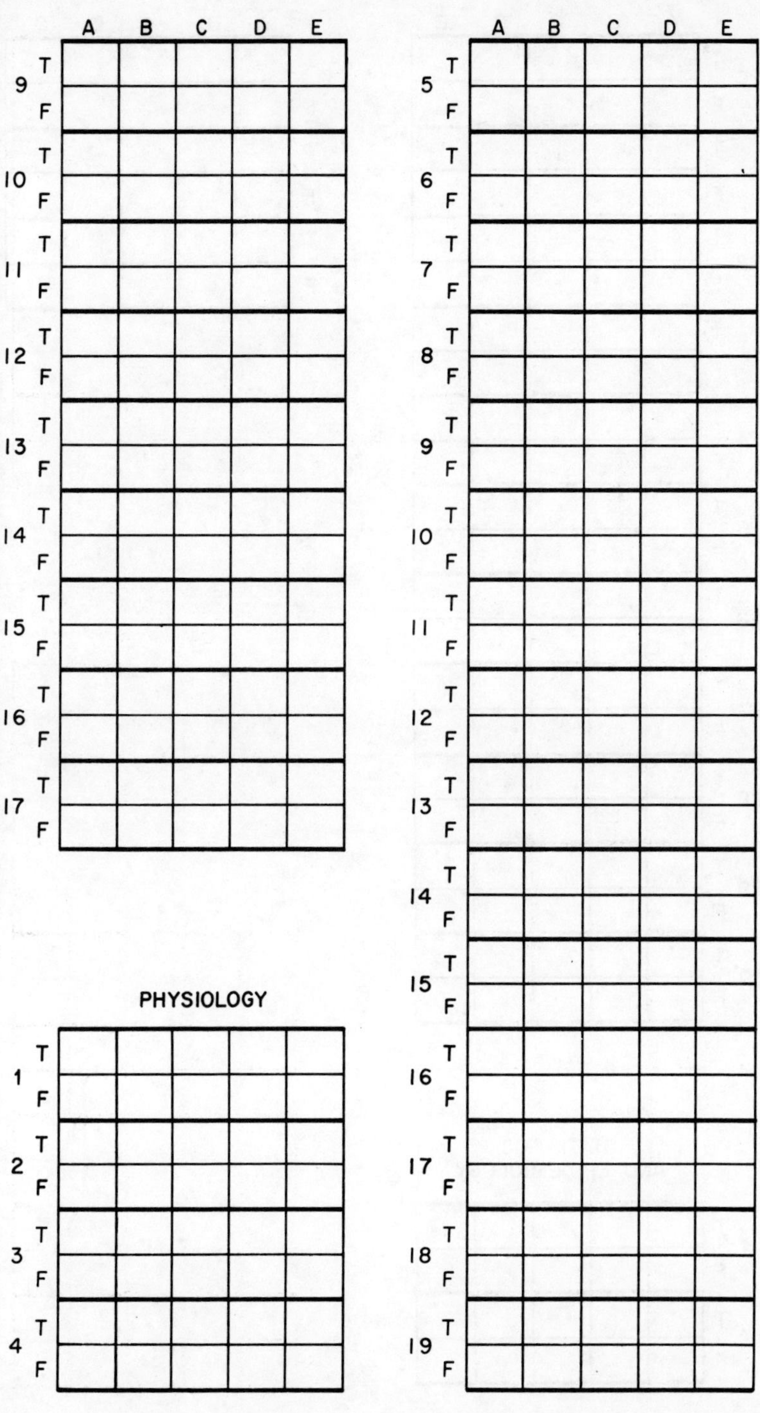

		A	B	C	D	E
9	T					
	F					
10	T					
	F					
11	T					
	F					
12	T					
	F					
13	T					
	F					
14	T					
	F					
15	T					
	F					
16	T					
	F					
17	T					
	F					

PHYSIOLOGY

1	T					
	F					
2	T					
	F					
3	T					
	F					
4	T					
	F					

		A	B	C	D	E
5	T					
	F					
6	T					
	F					
7	T					
	F					
8	T					
	F					
9	T					
	F					
10	T					
	F					
11	T					
	F					
12	T					
	F					
13	T					
	F					
14	T					
	F					
15	T					
	F					
16	T					
	F					
17	T					
	F					
18	T					
	F					
19	T					
	F					

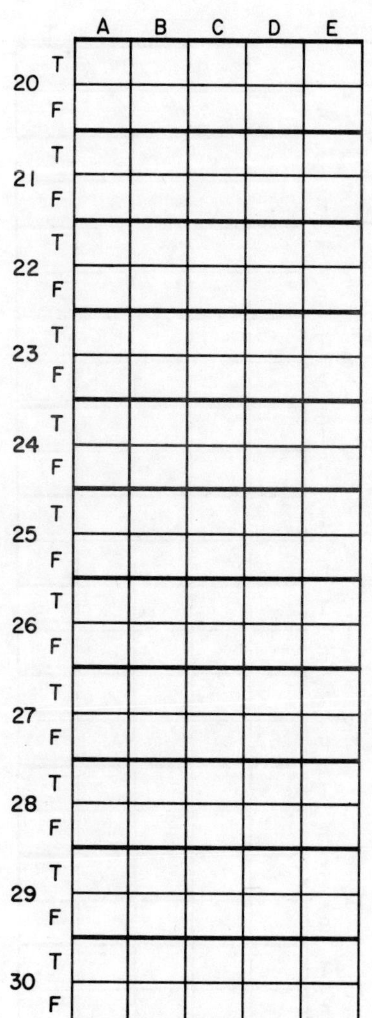

STATISTICS AND EPIDEMIOLOGY

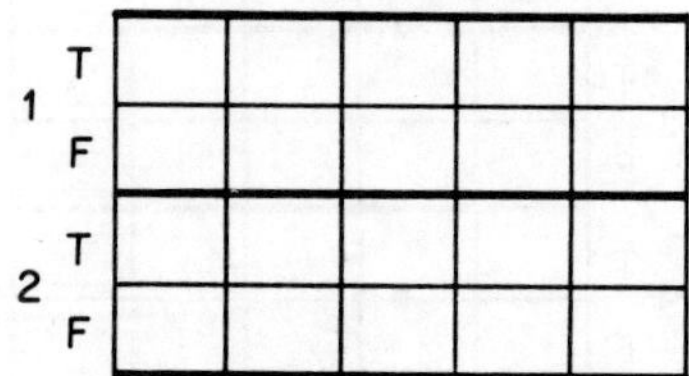

		A	B	C	D	E
3	T					
	F					
4	T					
	F					
5	T					
	F					

SECOND SERIES

CONTENTS

PREFACE

Examinations involving multiple choice questions have become a familiar pattern of examination for undergraduates and postgraduates. The purpose of this book is to explain simply and clearly what is involved in MCQ examinations in the basic science subjects. It also allows the potential candidate to familiarise him or herself with the type of question asked and the fields covered as well as to test their own capabilities and areas of weakness. The book is principally directed to the Part 1 examination for membership of the Royal College of Obstetricians and Gynaecologists, but it is applicable, too, to other similar examinations.

V. R. Tindall, 1985

INTRODUCTION

The purpose of this Tutor Book, as in the first series, is principally to aid teaching and learning. While it is aimed at helping potential obstetricians and gynaecologists, many of the sections will benefit other postgraduates.

The subjects covered are those required for the Part 1 MRCOG, and equivalent examinations, namely: anatomy, biochemistry, cell biology, embryology, endocrinology, elementary statistics and epidemiology, genetics, immunology, microbiology, pathology, pharmacology and physiology. In multiple choice questions (MCQs) there is often an overlap of subject material within an individual question, but the section under which a question is entered is related to the majority of the items. The questions have been grouped into batches of 20, in a manner similar to that of the Part 1 MRCOG examination itself. If three of these batches of 20 questions are taken together, they would be equivalent to one Part 1 MRCOG paper.

The majority of the questions or parts of the questions have been used under examination circumstances and have been amended according to their performance. It is hoped that by providing answers and comments this book will prove as useful as the previous volume in the process of learning or re-learning the techniques of answering multiple choice questions. It must again be stressed that no book of MCQs, even with answers, should be taken in isolation; it must be used in conjunction with the appropriate textbooks.

Answer sheets are included at the back of the book, so that the reader can complete them before looking at the answers, if so wished. Each question starts with an initial statement or word (stem), followed by five possible completions (items). All answers are (or should be) equally possible and do not include any mutually exclusive items. The reader has to decide, wherever possible, which items are true and which are false. For marking purposes, the reader should allocate one mark (+1) for the appropriate correct answer. One mark should be deducted (−1) for each incorrect answer. No mark (0) is to be awarded where no attempt has been made to answer an individual item. In each of the questions, any number of items may be correct, although in this book, as in examinations, relatively few questions will have all five items correct, and rarely will all five items be incorrect.

Since each of the 12 sections contains 20 questions, each with five parts, there are 100 potential marks to be gained for every section. Candidates should aim to gain an overall mark of 60 or 65 to pass the particular section at their first attempt. For each successive attempt the pass mark should be raised by 5–10 marks. Since candidates in the Part 1 MRCOG are informed whether they pass, fail or are borderline for a particular section, a mark of 55–59 (if 60 is taken as the pass mark) or 60–64 (if 65 is taken as the pass mark) would be regarded as a borderline grade. A mark of either 54 or less, or 59 or less, respectively, would be a fail grade. If three sections are taken together (that is equivalent to a 60-MCQ paper), then the appropriate pass standard would be a mark between 180 and 195. Analysis of the reader's performance in the three sections may give an idea of how to compensate for a borderline or fail grade in one or two sections. This will only be possible if the appropriate overall mark is reached.

The design of the sections has been deliberate in that 1–3 and 4–6 could represent, respectively, Paper 1 and Paper 2 of a Part 1 examination and, similarly, so could sections 7–9 and 10–12, thus allowing the reader the equivalent of two examinations. If sections 1–3 are paired with 10–12 and 4–6 with 7–9, the equivalent of another two examinations is also possible. As most doctors in training have limited periods of time available, the appropriate allocation of time for each section of 20 questions is 40 minutes.

Despite the criticism of the format of examinations, they are still a necessary hurdle in medicine. It is hoped that this book will help potential candidates in their ability to present their factual information in the MCQ format.

ACKNOWLEDGEMENTS

I would like to thank Professor J. Joseph, Professor of Anatomy, and Professor R. J. Pepperwell, Professor of Obstetrics and Gynaecology, who, after looking at the preliminary text, forwarded suggestions enabling me to verify certain questions and answers.

I would also like to thank Jane Holt and Wendy Wyatt, the two secretaries who typed this book from written manuscript.

1. ANATOMY AND EMBRYOLOGY

1.01 In the fetal skull at birth.
- **A.** The mastoid process is undeveloped.
- **B.** The great cerebral vein opens into the straight sinus of the dura mater.
- **C.** The anterior lobe of the pituitary gland is derived from a downgrowth of neural ectoderm.
- **D.** The bones of the base of the skull are fused.
- **E.** There are six fontanelles.

1.02 Muscles attached to the central tendon of the perineum (perineal body) include the:
- **A.** levator ani.
- **B.** sphincter urethrae.
- **C.** external anal sphincter.
- **D.** deep transverse perinei.
- **E.** ischiocavernosus.

1.03 The main supports of the uterus include the:
- **A.** round ligaments.
- **B.** cardinal (lateral cervical, Mackenrodt's) ligaments.
- **C.** broad ligaments.
- **D.** transverse perineal muscles.
- **S.** levator ani muscles.

Answers overleaf

1.01 A, B, D, E.
The mastoid process grows and develops in infancy and early childhood. The straight sinus is formed by the union of the great cerebral vein with the inferior saggital sinus. The anterior lobe of the pituitary gland is derived from the ectodermal roof of the stomodeum, the posterior lobe is derived from the floor of the diencephalon.

1.02 A, B, C, D.
Several muscles converge on the central tendon in the female – the anterior fibres of the two levatores ani, the sphincter urethrae, the paired deep and superficial transverse perinei muscles, the anterior fibres of the external anal sphincter and the paired bulbospongiosus. The ischiocavernosus arises from the inner aspect of the tuberosity of the ischium behind the crus of the clitoris and from the adjacent portion of the ramus of the ischium. The muscle ends in an aponeurosis which is inserted into the sides and inferior surface of the crus. Its action is to compress the crura of the clitoris and retard the return of blood, thus serving to maintain the erection of the clitoris.

1.03 B, D, E.
The main supports of the uterus are its connective tissue ligaments – lateral cervical, uterosacral, pubocervical, all of which are attached to the cervix. The levatores ani also support the uterus. The rest of the uterine ligaments – round, broad, ovarian, if intact, do not prevent prolapse if the connective tissue ligaments, especially the lateral cervical and levatores ani are torn. The round ligament may be shortened in order to correct a retroverted uterus to a position of anteversion.

1.04 The uterine (Fallopian) tube:

A. does not undergo changes during the menstrual cycle.
B. has an ampulla which is its longest portion.
C. is developed from the paramesonephric duct.
D. is lined by a continuous columnar ciliated epithelium.
E. has an isthmus which contains more muscle proportionately than any other part of the extra uterine tube.

1.05 At birth the:

A. thymus is well developed.
B. temporal bone consists of four separate parts.
C. facial nerve lies deep to the mastoid process.
D. mandible is in two parts.
E. adrenal cortex is proportionately larger than in the adult.

1.06 The pudendal nerve:

A. leaves the pelvis through the lesser sciatic foramen.
B. lies in the lateral wall of the ischiorectal fossa.
C. gives off the inferior rectal nerve.
D. supplies branches to the internal anal sphincter.
E. supplies the superficial and deep perineal muscles.

1.07 The round ligament of the uterus:

A. raises a ridge on the anterior (inferior) layer of the broad ligaments.
B. passes into the inguinal canal.
C. contains the cremaster muscle.
D. is derived from the gubernaculum.
E. is continuous with the ovarian ligament at the cornua of the uterus.

Answers overleaf

1.04 B, C, E.
The whole of the genital tract, particularly the epithelial surface, undergoes cyclical changes during the reproductive phase of a woman's life. In item D, the important word is *continuous* – columnar ciliated epithelium is not continuous throughout. The tubal mucosa is composed of both ciliated and secretory cells.

1.05 A, B, D, E.
The facial nerve is relatively superficial because the mastoid process does not grow until infancy and early childhood. The temporal bone consists of four parts: the squamous part, the petrous (later petromastoid), the tympanic part and the styloid process.

1.06 B, C, E.
The pudendal nerve passes between the piriformis and the coccygeus muscles and leaves the pelvis through the lower part of the greater sciatic foramen. The inferior rectal nerve supplies branches to the external anal sphincter. The internal anal sphincter consists of smooth muscle and is supplied by the autonomic nervous system.

1.07 A, B, D, E.
Although the ligament of the ovary and the round ligament are both derived from the gubernacular cord, the ovarian ligament is attached to the back of the uterus and the round ligament to the front, inferior to the uterine tube. The cremaster muscle covers the spermatic cord in the male and the round ligament in the inguinal region. Therefore, the cremaster muscle is outside the round ligament as it passes through the inguinal canal.

1.08 In the anterior abdominal wall:

A. the inferior attachment of the rectus abdominis muscle is to the posterior surface of the pubic bone.
B. the pyramidalis muscle lies within the rectus sheath.
C. the rectus sheath has a posterior layer extending to the symphysis pubis.
D. the tendenous intersections of the rectus abdominis muscle are attached to the posterior layer of the rectus sheath.
E. the conjoint tendon blends medially with the anterior layer of the rectus sheath.

1.09 In relation to the conduction system of the normal heart:

A. the impulse originates in the atrioventricular (A-V) node.
B. the A-V node is situated in the wall of the coronary sinus.
C. the impulse spreads directly from atrial to ventricular muscle.
D. the A-V bundle lies in the interventricular septum.
E. the A-V bundle branches to supply each ventricle.

1.10 With regard to the development of the kidney and ureter:

A. the metanephros becomes the permanent kidney.
B. the ureteric bud arises from the ventral aspect of the metanephric duct.
C. the metanephric cap invests the renal pelvis.
D. the major calyces are formed from the ureteric bud.
E. the kidney ascends in a cranial direction.

1.11 The pudendal nerve:

A. arises from L2, 3 and 4.
B. passes through the greater sciatic foramen.
C. passes through the lesser sciatic foramen.
D. gives off the inferior rectal nerve.
E. gives off the dorsal nerve of the penis.

Answers overleaf

1.08 B, E.
The rectus abdominis muscle is attached inferiorly by two tendons. The lateral is attached to the crest of the pubis and may extend beyond the pubic tubercle. The medial merges with the muscle of the opposite side and is connected to the ligamentous fibres on the front of the symphysis pubis. The rectus muscle is attached superiorly to the cartilages of the 5th, 6th and 7th ribs. There is no posterior layer of the rectus sheath inferiorly. The tendenous intersections are attached to the anterior layer of the rectus sheath.

1.09 D, E.
It is generally believed that the impulse of a cardiac contraction, which originates in the S-A node, is conducted to both atria directly to reach the A-V node and then transmitted to the ventricles by the A-V node, the bundle of His and its limbs with their terminal ramifications. The A-V node itself lies above the orifice of the coronary sinus, embedded in the myocardial fibres of the atrial septum.

1.10 A, C, D, E.
Three successive renal systems appear in man. They are the pronephros and mesonephros, which are vestigial in man, and the metanephros which becomes the permanent kidney. The ureteric bud arises from the dorsal aspect of the mesonephric duct, close to the point of entry of the duct into the cloaca. The ureteric bud divides repeatedly to form successive generations of collecting tubules which in turn form the major calyces, the minor calyces and finally the collecting tubules of the kidney. At first, the kidneys lie in front of the sacrum. The intermediate mesoderm contributes to the metanephric cap so that renal enlargement occurs in a cranial direction. The kidneys attain their adult position during the eighth week of fetal life.

1.11 B, C, D, E.
The pudendal nerve arises from the anterior divisions of sacral nerves 2, 3 and 4.

1.12 In the normal human pelvis:

A. the promontory of the sacrum is the upper anterior border of the first sacral vertebra.
B. the anterior part of the sacrum has four paired foramina.
C. the joint between the two pubic bones is a synovial joint.
D. the acetabular fossa is wholly formed from parts of the pubic and ischial bones.
E. the transverse diameter of the brim is greater than the anteroposterior diameter.

1.13 The pleura:

A. is in contact with parietal and visceral structures.
B. extends into the interlobal fissures.
C. extends into the neck above the lateral third of the clavicle.
D. lies posterior to the upper pole of the right kidney.
E. receives sensory innervation from the phrenic nerve.

1.14 The nerve supply of the bladder:

A. contains parasympathetic motor fibres to the detrusor muscle.
B. contains sympathetic inhibitor fibres to the sphincter vesicae.
C. passes under the posterolateral extension of the transverse cervical ligaments.
D. has sympathetic sensory fibres which reach the spinal cord via the 2nd, 3rd and 4th sacral nerves.
E. has visceral afferent fibres associated with the hypogastric sympathetic plexuses.

Answers overleaf

1.12 A, B, E.
Most joints of the body, including all the joints of the limbs, belong to the synovial type of joint, with the exception of the tibio-fibular syndesmosis (fibrous joint) and the pubic symphysis which is a secondary cartilagenous joint. All three elements of the hip bone, namely the ilium, pubis and ischium, contribute to the formation of the acetabulum, although not in equal portions.

1.13 A, B, D, E.
The extension of the cervical pleura reaches above the medial (not lateral) third of the clavicle and posteriorly reaches as high as the lower edge of the neck of the first rib. It can be represented as a curved line drawn from the sternoclavicular joint to the junction of the medial and middle thirds of the clavicle, with the summit of the curve 2.5 cm above the clavicle.

1.14 A, C, E.
The postganglionic parasympathetic nerves are motor to the detrusor muscle and inhibitor to the sphincters. The postganglionic sympathetic fibres are motor to the sphincter vesicae, not inhibitory. The parasympathetic sensory fibres reach the spinal cord via the 2nd, 3rd and 4th sacral nerves, and the sympathetic fibres reach the cord via the 1st and 2nd lumbar nerves.

.15 The paramesonephric (Mullerian) ducts:
A. fuse to form the uterus.
B. form the ductus (vas) deferens.
C. are suppressed by the developing testis.
D. open into the urogenital sinus.
E. if maldeveloped produce an ectopia vesicae.

.16 With regard to the spinal cord and its coverings.
A. The spinal cord ends at the lower border of the 1st lumbar vertebra.
B. The cauda equina is composed of coccygeal nerve roots.
C. The dura mater ends at the level of the 2nd sacral vertebra.
D. The cerebrospinal fluid is not found below the level of the 4th lumbar vertebra.
E. The extradural (epidural) space lies between the dura and arachnoid mater.

.17 In veins:
A. there are sympathetic nerves.
B. the blood flow fluctuates with the pulse.
C. the blood flow in the venae cavae is increased during expiration.
D. there is elastic tissue similar to arteries.
E. there are valves.

.18 Branches from the posterior trunk of the internal iliac artery include the:
A. obturator artery.
B. inferior vesical artery.
C. internal pudendal artery.
D. middle rectal artery.
E. superior gluteal artery.

Answers overleaf

1.15 A, C, D.
The ductus (vas) deferens is formed from the mesonephric duct. In ectopia vesicae the anterior abdominal wall and the bladder do not develop; the child is born with the inside of the bladder, ureteric and urethral orifices exposed on the surface.

1.16 A, C.
The cauda equina consists of a sheaf of roots of lumbar, sacral and coccygeal nerves. The chosen site for lumbar puncture is between the spines of the 3rd and 4th, or 4th and 5th lumbar vertebrae and because the subarachnoid space extends CSF must be present as far as the 2nd sacral vertebra. The epidural space is outside the dura mater.

1.17 A, B, D, E.
The blood flow in the venae cavae is reduced during expiration.

1.18 E.
The branches of the posterior trunk are the iliolumbar, lateral sacral and superior gluteal arteries. The other arteries arise from the anterior trunks of the internal iliac artery.

1.19 The trachea:

A. is palpable in the neck.
B. is stretched during inspiration.
C. crosses anterior to the aortic arch.
D. is crossed by the isthmus of the thyroid gland.
E. receives an innervation from the phrenic nerves.

1.20 In the development of the female urogenital system:

A. endodermal elements are involved in vaginal development.
B. the ureter arises as an upgrowth from the lower part of the mesonephric duct.
C. the phallic portion of the urogenital sinus gives rise to the female urethra.
D. development of the mesonephric ducts in the male is inhibited by androgens.
E. the paired genital folds give rise to the labia minora.

Answers overleaf

1.19 A, B, D.
The aortic arch is in front of the trachea. The tracheal innervation is from the recurrent laryngeal nerves, vagi and sympathetic trunks.

1.20 A, B, E.
The phallic part of the urogenital sinus and the urogenital groove remain open as the vestibule in the female. Testicular androgens promote the continued growth of the mesonephric ducts and the masculinisation of the external genitalia, and they suppress the paramesonephric ducts.

2. ENDOCRINOLOGY AND STATISTICS

2.01 Human chorionic gonadotrophin:

A. has a luteinising effect on the ovarian follicle.
B. production is greatest in the first 3 months of pregnancy.
C. cross-reacts with luteinising hormone in immunoassays.
D. is present in amniotic fluid.
E. is a polypeptide hormone.

2.02 The hypothalamus produces releasing factors directly or indirectly for:

A. adrenocorticotrophic hormone.
B. parathormone.
C. glucagon.
D. testosterone.
E. thyroxine.

2.03 In the luteal phase of a normal menstrual cycle, there is an increase in the:

A. progesterone level in blood.
B. body temperature.
C. subnuclear vacuolation in the endometrial glands.
D. oestrogen level in blood.
E. luteinising hormone level in blood.

2.04 Testosterone:

A. depresses pituitary secretion of luteinising hormone.
B. promotes union of long bone epiphyses.
C. is a polypeptide.
D. is responsible for differentiation of male external genitalia.
E. is largely bound to a plasma globulin.

Answers overleaf

2.01 A, B, C, D.
HCG is a glycoprotein.

2.02 A, D, E.
The hypothalamic releasing hormones include thyrotoxin-releasing hormone, gonadotrophin-releasing hormone, growth hormone-releasing hormone and melanocyte-stimulating hormone-releasing hormone, and affect the release of the appropriate pituitary hormone. There are also release-inhibiting hormones.

2.03 A, B, C, D.
Mean LH levels vary very little during the menstrual cycle, except in the ovulation stage.

2.04 A, B, D, E.
Testosterone is a steroid hormone, a C-19 derivative. It is synthesised by the interstitial cells of the testes from cholesterol through pregnenolone, progesterone and hydroxyprogesterone, which is then converted to the C-19 ketosteroid, androstenedione, the immediate precursor of testosterone.

2.05 A normal (Gaussian) distribution of values:

A. has half its values below the first quartile.
B. has a mean identical to the mode.
C. has a median equal to the mean.
D. is symmetrical about the mode.
E. is necessary for the accurate calculation of standard deviation.

2.06 Thyroxine:

A. is synthesised from two tyrosine units and three atoms of iodine.
B. circulates as free thyroxine.
C. levels in the blood are elevated during pregnancy.
D. is essential for adequate red cell production.
E. is slower in its action than triiodothyronine.

2.07 Oestrogens:

A. are responsible for the development of the vulva and vagina at puberty.
B. are responsible for growth of body hair.
C. cause deposition of glycogen in vaginal epithelium.
D. cause pigmentation of the areola of the breasts.
E. are produced by the corpus albicans.

2.08 Prolactin:

A. is secreted in the hypothalamus.
B. is necessary for mammary duct growth.
C. secretion is controlled by an inhibiting factor from the hypothalamus.
D. plasma levels are unaffected by pregnancy.
E. is identical with placental lactogen.

Answers overleaf

2.05 B, C, D, E.
In a normal distribution, half the values would be above and half would be below the mean, mode and median.

2.06 C, D, E.
Thyroxine (T4) has four atoms of iodine; over 99% of circulating thyroid hormones are protein bound.

2.07 A, C, D.
Growth of hair in the female is primarily due to androgens rather than oestrogens. The androgens come from the adrenal cortex and to a lesser extent from the ovaries.

2.08 C.
Prolactin is secreted from the anterior pituitary gland and the level increases in pregnancy. Prolactin is a protein similar in size and structure to growth hormone and placental lactogen, but it is not identical.

2.09 Which of the following may be used to assess adrenocortical function?
A. Urinary excretion of 17-oxosteroids.
B. Urinary excretion of 17-hydroxycorticosteroids.
C. Plasma cortisol level.
D. Urinary excretion of 5-hydroxy-indole acetic acid.
E. Urinary excretion of pregnanetriol.

2.10 Correlation coefficients:
A. are a measure of the association between two variables.
B. when positive, indicate that one event caused the other.
C. when positive, always indicate a statistically significant relationship between two variables.
D. can be calculated accurately from the slope of the line of best fit when the data are plotted graphically.
E. when negative, indicate that two variables are not related to each other.

2.11 Human growth hormone:
A. raises the plasma level of free (non-esterified) fatty acids.
B. reduces the urinary excretion of nitrogen.
C. causes an increased retention of calcium.
D. is produced by the basophil cells of the pituitary gland.
E. exhibits diurnal variation.

2.12 Parathormone:
A. increases the serum calcium level.
B. enhances reabsorption of calcium from bone.
C. is a polypeptide.
D. increases renal tubular reabsorption of phosphate.
E. has a direct effect on the absorption of calcium from the jejunum.

Answers overleaf

2.09 A, B, C, E.
Most serotonin is metabolised by oxidative deaminisation to 5-hydroxy indole acetic acid (the enzymc which catalyses this reaction is monoamine oxidase), and is usually conjugated with sulphates when present in the urine. It does not have any role in assessing adrenocortical function.

2.10 A, C.
The correlation coefficient is measured on a scale +1 through 0 to −1. Complete correlation between two variables is expressed by 1. When one variable increases as the other decreases, the correlation is positive; when one decreases as the other increases, it is negative. Correlation coefficients are calculated from the data using a special formula which can be found in any book of statistics. (It has not been the practice to expect candidates to know this formula and therefore it is not given here.)

2.11 A, B, C.
Growth hormone (and prolactin) is secreted from the eosinophil cells of the anterior pituitary gland. Normally, basal circulating levels of growth hormone occur during the day, with increased secretion during the first hours of sleep.

2.12 A, B, C.
One of the main actions of parathormone is to reduce renal tubular reabsorption of phosphate. The absorption of calcium from the jejunum requires the production of a Ca-binding transport protein in the mucosal cell. Formation of this protein is controlled by the level of 1,25-dihydroxycholecalciferol (DHCC). Parathormone modulates the effect of DHCC as an increase in parathormone increases the activity of an enzyme in the kidney, thereby producing more DHCC.

.13 Human ovulation:
A. is initiated by follicle-stimulating hormone.
B. occurs within 36 hours of the luteinising hormone peak.
C. is preceded by a marked rise in blood progesterone.
D. may occur during breast-feeding.
E. may be stimulated by undernutrition.

.14 Aldosterone:
A. promotes retention of sodium by the kidney.
B. potentiates the pressor effect of noradrenaline.
C. excretion is increased in proportion to circulating progesterone.
D. production increases when blood volume expands.
E. promotes gluconeogenesis.

.15 Statistics.
A. The standard deviation is the square root of the variance.
B. The range of results is the difference between the highest and the lowest values.
C. In a normal distribution curve, the mean value ±1 standard deviation (SD) contains 66% of the results.
D. In an even set of numbers the median value is the average of the middle two numbers.
E. If a frequency distribution curve is bimodal, it usually means that the group is homogeneous.

.16 Antidiuretic hormone (arginine vasopressin):
A. is a peptide.
B. is secreted at a rate determined by plasma osmolarity.
C. increases the permeability of the cells of the renal collecting duct to water.
D. is secreted by nerve cells with their cell bodies in the hypothalamus.
E. affects the blood pressure by a direct action on the baroreceptors.

Answers overleaf

2.13 B, D.
Ovulation is triggered by the pre-ovulatory surge of LH. Progesterone levels rise after ovulation. In general, undernutrition is associated with anovulation.

2.14 A, B, C.
Aldosterone production is reduced when the blood volume expands. Its secretion is controlled by the electrolyte mechanism, and the renin–angiotensin system. Cortisol promotes gluconeogenesis; aldosterone is involved in the homoeostasis of sodium and potassium.

2.15 A, B, C, D.
A bimodal frequency distribution curve would be associated with a heterogeneous group, or would contain at least two different groups.

2.16 A, B, C, D.
The pressor effect of vasopressin is of no significance under normal circumstances. Large changes in plasma volume also influence the ADH secretion. The baroreceptors may send stimuli to the hypothalamus via the vagus nerves but there is no direct effect of ADH on the baroreceptors.

.17 Progesterone:
- **A.** is responsible for the development of secondary sex characteristics.
- **B.** is an intermediate product in the synthesis of adrenocortical hormones.
- **C.** increases the output of sodium.
- **D.** is predominantly excreted as pregnanetriol.
- **E.** is synthesised from cholesterol.

.18 The thyroid gland:
- **A.** is normally stimulated by long-acting thyroid stimulator.
- **B.** stores colloid within its epithelial cells.
- **C.** enlarges in pregnancy.
- **D.** is stimulated by a posterior pituitary hormone.
- **E.** actively traps inorganic iodine from plasma.

.19 In congenital adrenal cortical hyperplasia:
- **A.** the commonest cause is a deficiency of C-21 hydroxylase.
- **B.** plasma cortisol is raised.
- **C.** urinary excretion of 17-oxosteroids is elevated.
- **D.** acute Addisonian crisis may occur.
- **E.** the karyotype is abnormal.

.20 Epidemiology and statistics.
- **A.** The incidence of a disorder indicates the proportion of a population suffering from it at any one time.
- **B.** The time incidence of a disease may be calculated from the number of new cases occurring each year in a defined population.
- **C.** In describing the specific epidemiological characteristics of a population with a condition, the total rate is the ratio:

$$\frac{\text{all cases in the population}}{\text{total number of the population}}$$

- **D.** The prevalence of a disease is the number of new cases in a stated period of time.
- **E.** The standardised mortality ratio is the mortality rate of a specific group expressed as a percentage of the mortality rate of the total population.

Answers overleaf

2.17 B, C, E.
The body changes that develop in girls at puberty are in part due to oestrogens and in part simply to the absence of testicular androgens. Progesterone is predominantly excreted as pregnanediol.

2.18 C, E.
Thyroid-stimulating hormone (TSH) is secreted from the anterior pituitary gland. Long-acting thyroid stimulator (LATS) duplicates most actions of TSH but its maximal thyroid-stimulating effect occurs many hours after that of TSH, hence its name. LATS is an antibody developed as an autoimmune phenomenon against thyroid protein. Transplacental transfer of LATS from mother to fetus may be responsible for neonatal thyrotoxicosis. The thyroid gland consists of innumerable follicles, each consisting of a single layer of epithelial cells surrounding colloidal fluid.

2.19 A, C, D.
Since there is a block in the synthesis of cortisol, the plasma level of cortisol cannot be raised. The individual is a normal female or normal male, and the karyotype is therefore normal.

2.20 B, C, D, E.
The incidence is the rate of occurrence of new cases (or disorders) in a defined population in a period of time.

3. BIOCHEMISTRY

3.01 Vitamin D:

A. is water soluble.
B. is absorbed from the small intestine.
C. is present in citrus fruits.
D. is stored in the body fat.
E. is a sterol.

3.02 Iodine.

A. Inorganic iodine in plasma is excreted in urine.
B. The plasma level of inorganic iodine rises in pregnancy.
C. Inorganic iodine is actively trapped by the thyroid gland.
D. Inorganic iodine is actively trapped by the mammary gland.
E. Iodine trapping is stimulated by thyroid-stimulating hormone.

3.03 Calcium.

A. The concentration of the serum is normally 8.5–10 mg/100 ml (2.1–2.6 mmol/l).
B. Calcium is present in the body in larger amounts than any other cation.
C. It is 40–60% ionised.
D. It becomes less ionised when blood pH falls.
E. The serum calcium is characteristically raised in hyperthyroidism.

Answers overleaf

3.01 B, D, E.
Vitamin D is one of the fat-soluble vitamins and is present in eggs, butter, fortified margarine and fish. The term vitamin D is used to refer to a group of closely related steroids produced by the action of ultraviolet light on certain provitamins. There is no evidence that adults require vitamin D in their diet; infants, children, pregnant and lactating women require supplementary therapy.

3.2 A, C, D, E.
During pregnancy the renal clearance of iodide doubles, the plasma level inorganic iodide falls, and thyroid clearance of iodine rises to three times normal, enabling the absolute iodine uptake to remain within the normal range.

3.3 A, B, C, D, E.
All true.

3.04 Carbohydrate in food.

A. Starch is a glucose polysaccharide.
B. Sucrose is a disaccharide of glucose and fructose.
C. Cellulose is a fructose polysaccharide.
D. Dietary carbohydrate is oxidised in the body to carbon dioxide and water.
E. Maltose is a disaccharide of glucose and fructose.

3.05 The rate of transfer of a substance into a cell:

A. by passive diffusion depends on the relative concentrations on the two sides of the cell wall.
B. by passive diffusion is the same for stereo-isomers.
C. by active transport is dependent on molecular size.
D. by active transport is usually more rapid for the naturally occurring isomer.
E. by active transport has a fixed upper limit.

3.06 Uric acid:

A. is the principal end-product of purine metabolism in man.
B. is excreted in the bile.
C. is derived from nucleoproteins.
D. excretion in urine is reduced by the administration of corticosteroid therapy.
E. is highly soluble in body fluids.

3.07 Folic acid is:

A. involved in purine synthesis.
B. essential for desoxyribonucleic acid (DNA) synthesis.
C. co-enzyme A.
D. heat stable.
E. involved in the tricarboxylic acid (Krebs') cycle.

Answers overleaf

3.4 A, B, D.
Cellulose, the chief constituent of the framework of plants, consists of long chains of β-D-glucopyranose units, i.e. is a glucose polysaccharide. Maltose is a disaccharide of glucose only.

3.5 A, B, D, E.
Active transport requires the active expenditure of chemical energy (work) and establishes, or maintains, a gradient. It is not dependent on molecular size.

3.6 A, B, C.
Uric acid excretion is diminished when the diet has a low purine content, a low protein content, a low calorific value, or consists of fat rather than of carbohydrate. It is not affected by corticosteroid therapy. Uric acid is not very soluble in body fluids.

3.7 A, B.
Folic acid is water soluble and unstable to heat. It is not involved in the Krebs' urea cycle. Panothenic acid, not folic acid, is a constituent of co-enzyme A.

3.08 Insulin:

A. circulates in a free state in the blood.
B. secretion is increased by sulphonylureas.
C. can be synthesised.
D. stimulated lipogenesis.
E. is composed of chains of amino acids.

3.09 Energy metabolism.

A. The brain is responsible for 20% of basal energy consumption.
B. The basal metabolic rate (BMR) is related to body size.
C. The energy output of an average woman is 5000–6000 kilocalories (21–25 megajoules) per day.
D. the respiratory quotient equals the amount of CO_2 produced divided by the amount of O_2 consumed per minute.
E. Weight for weight, fat persons have a higher energy output than thin persons.

3.10 The serum alkaline phosphatase activity is characteristically raised in:

A. senile osteoporosis.
B. intrahepatic cholestasis.
C. extensive Paget's disease of bone.
D. osteomalacia.
E. metastatic prostatic carcinoma.

3.11 Vitamin B_{12}.

A. The maintenance of adequate stores depends upon the secretion of intrinsic factor by the stomach.
B. Absorption takes place throughout the small intestine.
C. Deficiency leads to a megaloblastic appearance of the bone marrow.
D. It is synthesised exclusively by bacteria.
E. It contains copper.

Answers overleaf

3.8 B, C, D, E.
Insulin circulates in the blood plasma bound to a β-globulin.

3.9 A, B, D.
The average energy expenditure of an average women is 1700–2900 kcal and for men 2400–4000 kcal. Both basal metabolic rate and energy expenditure of mechanical work are directly proportional to body weight.

3.10 B, C, D.
The alkaline phosphatase level is normal in osteoporosis. The acid, not alkaline, phosphatase level may be elevated in metastatic prostatic carcinoma.

3.11 A, C, D.
Absorption of vitamin B_{12} only takes place selectively in the ileum, compared with iron which is absorbed in the duodenum and upper duodenum. Vitamin B_{12} (or cyanocobalamin), consists of the corrin ring similar to the porphyrins that include a cobalt ion at their centre.

3.12 Creatinine:

A. is synthesised in the liver.
B. has a plasma clearance rate equivalent to the glomerular filtration rate.
C. is an end-product of purine metabolism.
D. plasma concentration is related to total muscle mass.
E. plasma concentration is raised in normal pregnancy.

3.13 A deficiency of the substrates concerned in energy production by the cell occurs in:

A. severe lack of dietary protein.
B. hypoxia.
C. obesity.
D. diminished food intake.
E. malabsorption.

3.14 Hypoglycaemia:

A. is associated with acinar cell tumours of the pancreas.
B. occurs when a normal person fasts for 48 hours.
C. is a recognised feature of untreated hyperthyroidism.
D. is a characteristic feature of induced hypothermia.
E. is associated with a rise in catecholamines.

3.15 Essential amino acids include:

A. glutamic acid.
B. leucine.
C. phenylalanine.
D. histidine.
E. arginine.

Answers overleaf

3.12 B, D.
Creatinine is formed largely in muscle. Creatine is synthesised in the liver from three amino acids and discharged into the blood and taken up by the muscles as required. In humans, the end-product of purine metabolism is uric acid. The plasma concentration of creatinine falls in pregnancy.

3.13 A, B, E.
Obesity is often divided into two types: one in which there is an increase in the amount of fat per fat cell, but no increase in the number of fat cells, and the other in which there is an increase in the number of fat cells as well. In obesity, there is no deficiency of the substrates. Providing the balance is correct, there would be no problem with diminished food intake.

3.14 E.
Hunger, and therefore fasting, will tend to raise, not lower, the blood sugar. Thyroxine increases the blood sugar and hyperthyroidism would not be associated with hypoglycaemia. It is not a characteristic feature of hypothermia; all metabolic and physiological processes slow down without adverse features.

3.15 B, C.
The amino acids which cannot be synthesised by the body in sufficient quality and quantity to fulfil its normal requirements are called essential amino acids. There are 8 essential amino acids for man, and the other six are valine, isoleucine, threonine, methionine, tryptophan and lysine.

3.16 Characteristic features of severe vitamin C deficiency.
A. Follicular hyperkeratosis.
B. Peripheral neuropathy.
C. Impaired wound healing.
D. Macrocytic anaemia.
E. Increased capillary fragility.

3.17 Glucagon:
A. is secreted by the beta-cells of the pancreatic islets.
B. is essential for the maintenance of the blood glucose level.
C. secretion rate is inversely proportional to the blood glucose level.
D. increases the breakdown of glycogen.
E. increases the breakdown of triglycerides.

3.18 Catecholamines are produced by:
A. the liver.
B. adrenergic nerves.
C. the central nervous system.
D. the spleen.
E. the adrenal gland.

3.19 Triglycerides:
A. are the major component of dietary fat.
B. consist of three fatty acids linked to glucose.
C. cross the placenta freely.
D. are carried in the plasma by lipoproteins.
E. have an increased plasma concentration during pregnancy.

3.20 Histamine:
A. is stored in basophil cells of the blood.
B. is stored in mast cells.
C. is an essential amino acid.
D. is released in response to tissue trauma.
E. blocks anaphylactoid reactions.

Answers overleaf

3.16 A, C, D, E.
Deficiency of vitamin C is not associated with peripheral neuropathy, which is connected with vitamin B deficiencies.

3.17 C, D, E.
The alpha, not beta, cells secrete glucagon. It stimulates phosphorylase activity in the liver, thereby increasing glycogenolysis. It also reduces intestinal motility and gastric secretion.

3.18 B, C, E.
Catecholamines are released from autonomic neurons and adrenal medullary cells.

3.19 A, D, E.
Triglycerides are formed from one molecule of glycerol and three molecules of fatty acids. Free fatty acids cross the placenta freely and their transfer rate is related to maternal plasma levels.

3.20 A, B, D.
Histamine is not an essential amino acid. (See question 3.15 and its answer for the list of essential amino acids.) The action of histamine resembles that of anaphylactic shock in various animal species.

4. PHYSIOLOGY

4.01 The duodenum secretes a hormone which:

A. causes a copious flow of pancreatic juice rich in bicarbonate.
B. decreases gastric motility.
C. is stimulated by products of fat digestion.
D. leads to a flow of pancreatic juice free of enzymes.
E. contains cyanocobalamin.

4.02 Carbon dioxide:

A. is carried in red blood cells as carboxyhaemoglobin.
B. in the blood increases the oxygen-binding power of haemoglobin.
C. entry into the red blood cells results in the movement of chloride ions into the erythrocytes.
D. partial pressure is greater in the systemic venous system than in the arterial system.
E. in arterial blood is predominantly in solution.

4.03 The respiratory centre:

A. is situated in the medulla oblongata.
B. is regulated by afferent vagal impulses.
C. ceases rhythmical activity if both vagi are cut.
D. responds to impulses from the cerebral cortex.
E. is sensitive to pH alteration in the blood.

4.04 Physiological changes during pregnancy.

A. The cardiac output increases.
B. The glomerular filtration rate decreases.
C. The plasma volume increases.
D. The red cell mass decreases.
E. The basal metabolic rate increases.

Answers overleaf

4.01 A, B, C, D.
Cyanocobalamin (vitamin B_{12}) is not a constituent of the duodenal hormones.

4.02 C, D.
Carbon dioxide forms carbaminohaemoglobin. It has no direct influence on the oxygen-binding power of haemoglobin. Factors which affect the oxygen–haemoglobin dissociation curve are pH, temperature and the concentration of 2,3 diphosphoglycerate. The pH of blood falls as its CO_2 content rises, so when the $P\text{co}_2$ rises, the curve shifts to the right, and the affinity of haemoglobin for oxygen is reduced. The bulk of the carbon dioxide is present as bicarbonate.

4.03 A, B, D, E.
The rhythmic discharge of neurons in the respiratory centre is spontaneous and modified by centres in the pons and afferents in the vagus nerves from receptors in the lung. It still continues actively, albeit at a different rate, if the vagi are cut.

4.04 A, C, E.
The glomerular filtration rate increases, as does the red cell mass.

4.05 Cerebrospinal fluid:

A. has a normal albumin content of 20 mg/100 ml.
B. has a $P\text{CO}_2$ higher than that of arterial blood.
C. has a specific gravity of 1.030 to 1.040.
D. is secreted from the choroid plexus.
E. volume is 50–60 ml in the average-sized adult.

4.06 Smooth muscle:

A. when stretched tends to depolarise and contract.
B. has cross striations.
C. contains actomyosin.
D. has an inherent rhythm.
E. develops from endoderm.

4.07 In the normal human kidney:

A. tubular reabsorption of hydrogen ions is an important mechanism for maintaining normal body pH.
B. tubular reabsorption of glucose occurs in the distal convoluted tubule.
C. tubular reabsorption of sodium is increased by aldosterone.
D. glomerular filtrate is formed by a process of ultrafiltration.
E. 50% of plasma entering the kidney is filtered.

4.08 Normal human seminal fluid:

A. coagulates *in vitro*.
B. contains sucrose.
C. has a pH of 4–5.
D. may contain up to 10–15% of morphologically abnormal spermatozoa.
E. originates mainly in the testes.

Answers overleaf

4.05 A, B, D.
The specific gravity is about 1·005 and the fluid is formed by the secretory activity of the epithelial cells of the choroid plexus of the intraventricular system. The content of CSF in humans is of the order of 130–150 ml.

4.06 A, C, D.
Cross striations are characteristic features of skeletal muscle. Muscles are derived from the mesoderm.

4.07 A, C, D.
Glucose, amino acids and bicarbonates are reabsorbed, together with sodium, in the proximal portion of the proximal tubule. The filtration fraction, i.e. the ratio of the glomerular filtration rate to the renal plasma flow, is normally 0.16–0.20.

4.08 A, D.
Seminal fluid contains fructose (1.5–6.5 mg/ml), not sucrose. It has a pH of 7.35–7.50. Sixty per cent of the volume is contributed from the seminal vesicles and 20% is from prostatic secretions.

4.09 Hyperventilation can cause:

A. a fall in plasma bicarbonate concentration.
B. an increase in urine output.
C. a reduction in cardiac output.
D. increased sensitivity to barbiturates.
E. tetany.

4.10 Arterial systolic blood pressure varies with:

A. arteriolar tone.
B. pulse rate.
C. blood viscosity.
D. oxygen lack.
E. posture.

4.11 Lung function.

A. The residual volume is the volume of gas in the lungs (excluding the anatomical dead space) at the end of maximum expiration.
B. The expiratory reserve is the volume which can be expired after the end of normal expiration.
C. Vital capacity is the volume of gas which can be inspired after normal expiration.
D. Tidal volume increases in pregnancy.
E. The minute volume is the tidal volume multiplied by the respiratory rate.

4.12 Which of the following substances are essential for normal erythropoiesis?

A. Folic acid.
B. Iodine.
C. Cyanocobalamin.
D. Zinc.
E. Pyridoxine.

Answers overleaf

4.09 A, D, E.
There is renal compensation for the respiratory alkalaemia which develops and there is predominantly an alkaline urine containing bicarbonate, but there is no increase in output. The cardiac output is raised by hyperventilation.

4.10 A, B, C, D, E.
All basic facts.

4.11 A, B, D, E.
Vital capacity is the maximal expiration preceded by a maximal inspiration.

4.12 A, C, E.
Iodine deficiency is associated with thyroid disorders and only indirectly may affect erythropoieses, since thyroxine and TSH stimulate erythropoiesis through an unknown action on erythropoietin production. It is so indirect that a false answer would be appropriate. Zinc deficiencies in humans cause skin ulcers, loss of hair and hypogonadal dwarfism.

.13 In the metabolism of iron:
- **A.** absorption occurs mainly in the duodenum and upper jejunum.
- **B.** absorption is increased when stores are depleted.
- **C.** traces of copper are essential for haemopoiesis.
- **D.** transferrin is increased in pregnancy.
- **E.** ferric salts are more readily absorbed than ferrous salts.

.14 Bile salts:
- **A.** are derived from cholesterol.
- **B.** are principally absorbed from the large intestine.
- **C.** are required for the absorption of vitamin D.
- **D.** stimulate the flow of bile when given orally.
- **E.** in excess give rise to steatorrhoea.

.15 Water intoxication is characterised by:
- **A.** epileptiform convulsions.
- **B.** headache.
- **C.** inhibition of antidiuretic hormone secretion.
- **D.** hypernatraemia.
- **E.** concentrated urine.

.16 The velocity of blood flow:
- **A.** in the capillaries is higher than in the arteries.
- **B.** in the veins is faster than in the venules.
- **C.** falls to about zero in the ascending aorta during diastole.
- **D.** in the pulmonary circulation is less than the velocity through the systemic circulation.
- **E.** in the placenta intervillous space is higher than through the uterine vessels.

Answers overleaf

4.13 A, B, C, D.
Ferrous salts are more readily absorbed than ferric salts.

4.14 A, C, D.
Ninety to ninety-five per cent of the bile salts are absorbed from the terminal ileum by an extremely active transport process. The remaining 5% enter the colon and are converted to deoxycholic acid and lithocholic acid. Lithocholate is relatively insoluble and mostly excreted in the faeces; deoxycholate is absorbed. Steatorrhoea is a condition in which an excess of split fat appears in the faeces, as in coeliac disease.

4.15 A, B, C.
There is a reduction of all plasma electrolytes and the plasma osmolality is decreased in water intoxication. The packed cell volume and plasma protein level are also reduced. The urine is diluted but not always of large volume. Whereas there may be an early diuresis, the renal cells will soon become damaged and oliguria or even anuria may follow.

4.16 B, C, D.
The velocity of blood flow is higher in arteries than in capillaries. Blood flow in the intervillous spaces is very sluggish compared with that in the uterine blood vessels.

.17 Starling's law of the heart:

A. states that the strength of myocardial contraction is a function of the initial length of the muscle fibres.
B. explains how stroke volume may be maintained when peripheral resistance rises.
C. explains the rise in the cardiac output in exercise when the end-diastolic volume of the ventricles is increased.
D. explains why the output of the left and right ventricles is equal in the long term.
E. explains the normal heart rate for the adult.

.18 In the stomach:

A. 20–25% of the products of ingested protein are absorbed.
B. production of hydrochloric acid depends on the activity of carbonic anhydrase.
C. fat increases gastric emptying.
D. there are oxyntic (parietal) cells.
E. there is a rich lymphatic supply.

.19 Brown fat:

A. is subcutaneous adipose tissue found in elderly people.
B. is richer in mitochondria than in ordinary adipose tissue.
C. increases its rate of heat production in response to stimulation of its sympathetic nerve supply.
D. is more important than shivering in neonatal thermoregulation.
E. is part of the physiological increase in maternal fat during pregnancy.

.20 Contraction of the diaphragm:

A. increases the anteroposterior diameter of the chest.
B. increases intra-abdominal pressure.
C. lowers intrapleural pressure.
D. in quiet respiration accounts for 70–75% of the change in intrathoracic volume.
E. is innervated by the vagus nerve.

Answers overleaf

4.17 A, B, C, D.
Starling's law of the heart is related to the mechanisms of contraction of the heart; it does not explain its normal rate. The heart rate is determined by the sinoatrial node and the various factors which influence its inherent rhythm.

4.18 B, D, E.
Protein digestion into polypeptides begins in the stomach but the bulk of the absorption is in the small intestine. Amino acid absorption is rapid in the duodenum and jejunum but slow in the ileum. Only about 2–5% of protein in the intestine escapes digestion and absorption. Fat depresses gastric secretion and gastic emptying (by releasing enterogasterone).

4.19 B, C, D.
Brown fat is characterised by a high content of mitochondria, cytochromes and a well-developed blood supply and is more common in infants. Metabolic emphasis is placed on oxidation of both glucose and fatty acids. It is very important in neonatal thermoregulation as it is a significant source of heat production.

4.20 B, C, D.
The diaphragm raises the thoracic cage, as well as depressing the abdominal contents, while the abdominal muscles do the opposite. It is supplied by the phrenic nerve.

5. PATHOLOGY AND IMMUNOLOGY

5.01 In β-thalassaemia:
A. the synthesis of haemoglobin A is defective.
B. fetal haemoglobin synthesis persists.
C. the plasma iron is reduced.
D. the red cell survival time is increased.
E. the mean cell haemoglobin concentration (MCHC) is raised.

5.02 Which of the following are associated with an increased incidence of atheroma?
A. Cirrhosis of the liver.
B. A diet high in unsaturated fats of vegetable origin.
C. Hypertension.
D. Diabetes mellitus.
E. Sedentary occupation.

5.03 Lymphocytes:
A. are less sensitive to irradiation than granulocytes.
B. are reduced in numbers by immunosuppressive therapy.
C. are formed in the spleen.
D. enter the circulation via the lymphatics.
E. are the precursors of platelets.

Answers overleaf

5.01 A, B.
The poor synthesis of haemoglobin in the homozygous state (thalassaemia major) causes the red cells to be very hypochromic and extreme leptocytosis is characteristic. The blood film resembles that in iron deficiency anaemia. There is a considerable increase in the amount of HbF and the main effects are those of a very severe haemolytic anaemia. In the heterozygous state (thalassaemia minor), there is a mild anaemia and a tendency to develop gallstones. The level of HbA_2 is increased, as also may be that of HbF. The plasma iron level is normal or increased.

5.02 C, D, E.
Cirrhosis of the liver is an end-stage condition as it can be the end-result of liver damage due to many causes, but it is not associated with an increased incidence of atheroma. Most authorities recognise that levels of β-lipoproteins (which include cholesterol) are elevated. Since a diet of unsaturated fats of vegetable origin would lower the plasma cholesterol level, the incidence would not be expected to increase.

5.03 B, C, D.
Lymphocytes are more sensitive to irradiation. Platelets are formed within the cytoplasm of the granular megakaryocyte and released into the circulation when the cell dies.

.04 Trophoblast disease.

A. A fetus may co-exist with hydatidiform mole.
B. There is epidemiologically an inverse relationship to anencephaly.
C. Hydatidiform mole is associated with theca-lutein ovarian cysts.
D. Choriocarcinoma is preceded by hydatidiform mole in over 75% of cases.
E. Choriocarcinoma occurs in either sex.

05 The alkaline phosphatase is elevated in:

A. Paget's disease of bone.
B. carcinoma of the prostate confined to the prostate.
C. osteosarcoma.
D. obstructive jaundice.
E. hyperthyroidism.

.06 An inappropriate secretion of which of the following may occur in a patient with carcinoma of the bronchus?

A. Adrenocorticotrophin.
B. Parathormone.
C. Oxytocin.
D. Thyroid-stimulating hormone.
E. Antidiuretic hormone.

.07 Radiation physics.

A. An electron has a greater mass than a proton.
B. A positron has the same charge as an electron.
C. A proton has a positive charge.
D. A neutron has almost the same mass as a proton.
E. The hydrogen nucleus is a neutron.

Answers overleaf

5.04 A, B, C, E.
The figure quoted for hydatidiform mole as a precursor of choriocarcinoma is about 50% of cases.

5.05 A, C, D.
The acid phosphatase is elevated in prostatic carcinoma, but in particular in metastases from prostatic carcinoma. Hyperparathyroidism is associated with a moderately raised alkaline phosphatase, but not hyperthyroidism.

5.06 A, B, D, E.
Oxytocin is the only one which has not been noted to be present in ectopic hormone secretion. Apart from the amines produced by the carcinoid type of tumour, all the hormones are of polypeptoid nature.

5.07 C, D.
The electron is much lighter than the proton; its mass is only 1/1840th of the mass of a proton. The proton is a heavy particle, carrying a positive charge, and the electron is a much lighter particle which carries a *negative* charge of exactly equal magnitude (but of opposite sign) to that of a proton. The simplest atom is that of hydrogen; it consists of a central nucleus comprised of one proton around which one electron moves in a shell or orbit.

5.08 Wound healing is delayed with:
- **A.** the presence of infection.
- **B.** the presence of dead tissue.
- **C.** a deficient dietary intake of calcium.
- **D.** previous external radiation to the area concerned.
- **E.** administration of adrenal steroids.

5.09 Chronic pyelonephritis may:
- **A.** cause renal failure.
- **B.** cause hypertension.
- **C.** occur when there is obstruction to the outflow of urine.
- **D.** cause polyhydramnios.
- **E.** result from blood-borne infection.

5.10 Neonatal jaundice is caused by:
- **A.** prenatal phenobarbitone therapy.
- **B.** glucose-6-phosphate dehydrogenase deficiency.
- **C.** maternal rhesus isoimmunisation.
- **D.** biliary duct atresia.
- **E.** ultraviolet phototherapy.

5.11 ABO blood group antigens:
- **A.** are attached to the haemoglobin molecule.
- **B.** contain mucopolysaccharides.
- **C.** are determined by genes carried by sex chromosomes.
- **D.** can be found in the saliva.
- **E.** are detectable in the amniotic fluid.

5.12 Fatty change in liver cells:
- **A.** occurs in starvation.
- **B.** occurs in gross obesity.
- **C.** causes necrosis.
- **D.** can occur if cell function is normal.
- **E.** results from an excess of lipotropic factors.

Answers overleaf

5.08 A, B, D, E.
There is no evidence that a diet deficient in calcium delays wound healing.

5.09 A, B, C, E.
In general, chronic pyelonephritis is associated with growth retardation, with all its associated problems.

5.10 B, C, D.
Prenatal phenobarbitone therapy has been used to reduce the incidence of neonatal jaundice, and phototherapy is a standard therapy for the reduction of jaundice in neonates.

5.11 B, D, E.
ABO antigens are polysaccharide in nature, possibly occurring in red blood cells as glycolipid, and owe their specificity to sugar and amino acid residues. They are carried by autosomes.

5.12 A, B, D.
Fatty change does not cause necrosis, although it may cause focal cytoplasmic degeneration. The liver is unable to metabolise fat unless there is an adequate supply of raw materials for the manufacture of lipoprotein. Substances which are necessary for this conversion are called lipotropic factors, and, in particular, choline is important. Without it, fatty acid cannot be converted to phospholipid, and therefore fatty acid in the form of neutral fat accumulates.

5.13 In inflammation, phagocytosis is carried out by:
A. polymorphonuclear leucocytes.
B. B-lymphocytes.
C. T-lymphocytes.
D. monocytes.
E. histiocytes.

5.14 Pulmonary embolism:
A. is followed by pulmonary hypertension in less than 30% of cases.
B. produces a fall in right atrial pressure.
C. results if air enters the systemic veins.
D. due to blood clot is more common in group O individuals.
E. due to blood clot has racial variation.

5.15 Which of the following factors predispose to the development of carcinoma of the large bowel?
A. Familial intestinal polyposus.
B. Ulcerative colitis.
C. Amoebic dysentery.
D. Endometriosis.
E. Villous papilloma of the rectum.

5.16 Haemochromatosis:
A. is more common in females.
B. predisposes to diabetes mellitus.
C. involves normal total iron binding capacity (TIBC) of plasma.
D. may be evoked by parenteral iron therapy were this to be given for the treatment of haemoglobinopathies.
E. predisposes to primary carcinoma of the liver.

Answers overleaf

5.13 A, D, E.
Lymphocytes are associated with all aspects of specific immunity; some (B-lymphocytes) are associated with humoral immunity and others (T-lymphocytes) with cell-mediated immunity.

5.14 A, C, E.
Right atrial pressure rises as a result of pulmonary embolism. The incidence of thromboembolism is reported to be three times greater in individuals of blood group A, B or AB than in those of group O.

5.15 A, B, E.
There is no association between amoebic dysentery or endometriosis and carcinoma of the colon.

5.16 B, D, E.
It more commonly affects men, women presumably being protected by menstruation. The concentration of transferrin in plasma is quantitated in terms of the total iron binding capacity of the plasma, which is normally a third saturated with iron. In haemochromatosis it is almost completely saturated.

5.17 An immune response:
A. involves synthesis of globulins.
B. may delay phagocytosis.
C. is associated with an immediate increase in the number of circulating polymorphonuclear leucocytes.
D. is the explanation for the development of rhesus haemolytic disease.
E. is mediated by small lymphocytes.

5.18 Tumours of germ cell origin include:
A. benign dermoid cystic teratoma.
B. granulosa cell tumour.
C. non-gestational choriocarcinoma.
D. seminoma.
E. Brenner tumour.

5.19 Which of the following aneurysms are paired with the appropriate pathogenesis?
A. Thoracic aortic aneurysm — atheroma.
B. Abdominal aortic aneurysm — tertiary syphilis.
C. Cerebral (Berry) aneurysm — development fault.
D. Retinal microaneurysm — diabetes.
E. Varicose aneurysm — trauma.

5.20 Giant cells are a histological feature of which of the following conditions?
A. Tuberculosis.
B. Lobar pneumonia.
C. Herpes virus infection.
D. Gummata.
E. Talc granulomata.

Answers overleaf

5.17 A, D, E.
There is no delay in phagocytosis, and there would be an increase in lymphocytes, not polymorphonuclear leucocytes.

5.18 A, C, D.
The granulosa cell and Brenner tumours are not of germ cell origin.

5.19 A, C, D, E.
The abdominal aorta is rarely attacked in syphilis.

5.20 A, C, D, E.
Lobar pneumonia is associated with an oedematous exudate containing macrophytes and a few polymorphs, and in the later process the alveoli are crowded with polymorphs and red cells and thereafter by degenerating and dead polymorphs.

6. MICROBIOLOGY AND PHARMACOLOGY

6.01 *Clostridium welchii (perfringens)* is:
A. an obligatory anaerobe.
B. a spore-bearing bacillus.
C. motile.
D. a causative organism of food poisoning.
E. capable of producing a lethal toxin.

6.02 Ophthalmia neonatorum is caused by:
A. *Neisseria gonorrhoeae.*
B. pneumococci.
C. *Treponema pallidum.*
D. Herpesvirus hominis — Type II.
E. *Trichomonas vaginalis.*

6.03 BCG innoculation:
A. if positive, results in regional node enlargement.
B. if positive, produces reaction within 1 week.
C. should be given intramuscularly.
D. is effective in the newborn.
E. uses live attenuated tubercle bacilli.

6.04 *Schistosoma mansoni*:
A. frequently affects the liver.
B. enters the body by the ova being swallowed in drinking water.
C. lives part of its cycle in certain snails.
D. commonly causes haematuria.
E. is common in the northern parts of South America.

Answers overleaf

6.01 A, B, D, E.
Clostridium welchii is the only one of the clostridial organisms which is non-motile. It is also an invariable inhabitant of the human bowel.

6.02 A, B.
The last three organisms are obviously incorrect. The condition is manifest as a prurulent discharge from an infant within 21 days of birth. The common organisms are gonococcal, streptococcal, pneumococcal or *Esch. coli*, or the infections may be mixed.

6.03 A, D, E.
Following intradermal (the chosen route) inoculation, a small nodule appears and is usually well established in about 3 weeks.

6.04 A, C, E.
It is a species which occurs over much of Africa and tropical America. The eggs, which have a lateral spine, are laid in venules of the large intestine and pass in faeces. Secondary hosts are freshwater snails. *Schistosoma haematobium* affects mainly the bladder and *S. mansoni* mainly the intestinal tract, but the infection may involve every organ of the body.

6.05 Group A haemolytic streptococci:

A. can be isolated from the throat in 5–15% of normal adults and children.
B. are commensals in the colon.
C. are cultural on blood agar.
D. are facultative anaerobes.
E. develop penicillin resistance.

6.06 Toxoplasmosis.

A. It is caused by a virus.
B. The acute infection is diagnosed by a complement fixation test.
C. The causative agent multiplies within cells of the reticuloendothelial system.
D. It may follow ingestion of infected meat.
E. If affected, the fetus may develop symptoms a few weeks after birth.

6.07 Virus diseases which may affect the fetus *in utero*.

A. Variola.
B. Varicella.
C. Cytomegalic inclusion.
D. Poliomyelitis.
E. Herpes genitalis — Type II.

6.08 Syphilis.

A. The incubation period is usually between 1 and 7 days.
B. It has an infectious secondary stage.
C. The primary stage is often unrecognised.
D. The Wassermann reaction becomes positive in the tertiary stage.
E. Condyloma acuminatum is characteristic of the secondary stage.

Answers overleaf

6.05 A, C, D.
The non-haemolytic *Streptococcus faecalis* is always present in the colon, but not Group A haemolytic streptococci. So far they are penicillin sensitive.

6.06 C, D, E.
Toxoplasmosis arises from infection with the small protozoon, *Toxoplasma gondii*. Serological testing for the specific Toxoplasma antibodies is the primary method of diagnosis. Ig-antibodies to Toxoplasma may be detected by conventional indirect fluorescent antibody test, which is the most widely available. Other more reliable tests are only available at a few reference laboratories. *T. gondii* is an intracellular parasite and, unlike most intracellular protozoa, can invade and multiply in any type of host cell except non-nucleated erythrocytes. Once born, the child may develop symptoms within a few weeks or at a later date.

6.07 A, B, C, D, E.
All basic facts.

6.08 B, C.
There is systemic dissemination before any local manifestation appears. The chancre appears 2–4 weeks after exposure to infection, and 1–3 weeks after the appearance of the chancre the WR and antitreponemal antibodies first appear in blood. Condylomata acuminata are due to viral infection.

6.09 *Trichomonas vaginalis*:
- **A.** is a flagellated protozoon.
- **B.** is an intracellular organism.
- **C.** is an obligatory anaerobe.
- **D.** reproduces by binary fission.
- **E.** is transmitted by sexual intercourse.

6.10 When maternal rubella occurs during the first 12 weeks of pregnancy:
- **A.** the incidence of fetal abnormalities is about 25%.
- **B.** the commonest abnormality is congenital pyloric stenosis.
- **C.** it is followed by a rise in the IgM titre level.
- **D.** it is accompanied by a lymphocytosis.
- **E.** rubella vaccine should be given immediately.

6.11 Tetracyclines:
- **A.** in therapeutic doses are bactericidal.
- **B.** are mainly excreted in the urine.
- **C.** may cause liver damage in pregnancy.
- **D.** are concentrated in the bile.
- **E.** depress protein anabolism.

6.12 Which of the following drugs are monoamine-oxidase inhibitors?
- **A.** Hydralazine (Apresoline).
- **B.** Phenelzine (Nardil).
- **C.** Iproniazid (Marsilid).
- **D.** Tranylcypromine (Parnate).
- **E.** Chlorpromazine (Largactil).

Answers overleaf

6.09 A, D, E.
It is protozoon and not an intracellular organism. It is a facultative anaerobe, i.e. it is not dependent on gaseous oxygen but prefers an atmosphere containing some oxygen.

6.10 A, C, D.
The usual abnormalities are heart lesions, cataract and deafness. Mental deficiency is not common. Rubella vaccine should not be given.

6.11 B, C, D, E.
Tetracyclines are bacteriostatic, although with intravenous injections weakly bactericidal blood levels can be achieved. Nerve damage is more likely with intravenous therapy if given in pregnancy.

6.12 B, C, D.
Monamine-oxidase inhibitors are used much less frequently than tricyclic and related antidepressants because of the dangers of dietary and drug interactions. Hydrallazine is a hypotensive and vasodilator agent. Chlorpromazine (Largactil) is a phenothiazene.

6.13 Which of the following substances cause uterine relaxation?

A. Atropine.
B. Halothane.
C. Morphine sulphate.
D. Amyl nitrite.
E. Ethyl alcohol.

6.14 Bromocriptine:

A. is a dopamine receptor agonist.
B. inhibits prolactin release.
C. promotes growth hormone release.
D. is an ergot derivative.
E. is oxytoxic.

6.15 Prostaglandin $F_2\alpha$:

A. is a naturally occurring polypeptide.
B. causes contraction of the pregnant uterus.
C. lowers the diastolic blood pressure.
D. synthesis is inhibited by aspirin.
E. causes water retention.

6.16 Which of the following statements are true of anti-hypertensive agents?

A. Guanethidine sulphate (Ismelin) blocks post-ganglionic sympathetic transmission.
B. Ganglion-blocking agents exert their maximal effect on blood pressure in the erect posture.
C. Reserpine causes a disseminated lupus-like state (with LE cells in the circulating blood).
D. Some male patients on guanethidine sulphate complain of inability to ejaculate.
E. Methyldopa acts as a ganglion blocking agent.

Answers overleaf

6.13 B, D, E.
Atropine and morphine sulphate have no direct effect on the uterus.

6.14 A, B, D.
It does not promote but inhibits growth hormone release, and it is not oxytoxic.

6.15 B, D.
Prostaglandins are modified fatty acids and are the result of enzymatic synthesis from arachidonic acid. According to circumstances, prostaglandins can cause smooth muscle (vascular, uterine, bronchial) to contract or relax. $F_2\alpha$ does not lower the blood pressure and does not cause water retention.

6.16 A, B, D.
Adverse effects with reserpine are quite common, but not the one stated. The following are recognised: lethargy and apathy, nasal stuffiness, gain in weight and diarrhoea. Dyspnoea not associated with cardiac failure occurs. Anaesthesia in patients taking reserpine, or within 2 weeks of stopping, may cause hypotension. With large doses an extrapyramidal syndrome (indistinguishable from parkinsonism) occurs, but it is reversible. Decreased libido and nightmares may occur. Epileptics have more fits, and peptic ulcers may be activated. Methyldopa probably acts primarily in the brainstem vasomotor centres. The chief clinically important advantage of methyldopa is that it interferes with homoeostatic reflexes less than do adrenic neuron blockers, i.e. the blood pressure is controlled equally whether the patient is supine, standing or exercising.

6.17 Which of the following drugs are ineffective when taken by mouth?
A. Probenecid.
B. Heparin.
C. Cyclophosphamide.
D. Suxamethonium chloride.
E. Methicillin.

6.18 Atropine given subcutaneously in therapeutic doses:
A. increases the resting heart rate.
B. produces vasodilatation of the skin.
C. reduces the flow of saliva.
D. produces overactivity of the small intestine.
E. reduces gastric secretion.

6.19 Vasopressin:
A. causes a water diuresis.
B. in therapeutic doses, raises the blood pressure.
C. secretion is stimulated by nicotine.
D. in therapeutic doses, causes intestinal colic.
E. secretion is stimulated by an increase in the osmotic pressure of blood supplying the hypothalamus.

6.20 Morphine:
A. causes cutaneous vasodilatation.
B. lowers blood pressure.
C. reduces tone of the intestinal muscle.
D. causes respiratory acidosis.
E. has anticonvulsant properties.

Answers overleaf

6.17 B, D.
Probenecid, cyclophosphamide and methicillin can be taken orally. Heparin is given subcutaneously or intravenously, and suxamethonium intravenously.

6.18 A, C.
Atropine has no significant effect on peripheral blood vessels in therapeutic doses, but in poisoning there is marked vasodilatation. Smooth muscle is relaxed and in the gastrointestinal tract there is reduction of tone and peristalsis. Whereas anticholinergic drugs are capable of reducing the total number of millimoles of hydrochloric acid secreted, this is not so with therapeutic doses given subcutaneously.

6.19 C, E.
It is antidiuretic. The official name is misleading, for only in large unphysiological or pharmacological doses does vasopressin cause contraction of all smooth muscle, raising the blood pressure and causing intestinal colic.

6.20 A, D.
Lowering of blood pressure may occur if patients are also taking anti-hypertensive drugs, but otherwise there is no such effect. Morphine acts directly on the smooth muscle of both large and small bowel, causing it to contract. Peristalsis is reduced and segmentation increased. Morphine has useful hypnotic effects but not anticonvulsant properties.

7. ANATOMY AND EMBRYOLOGY

7.01 The pelvic splanchnic nerves:

A. contain parasympathetic visceral motor nerves.
B. supply motor fibres to the descending colon.
C. supply vasodilator fibres to the erectile tissue of the clitoris.
D. form a plexus with branches of the sacral sympathetic ganglia.
E. originate from the ventral (anterior primary) rami of the 2nd, 3rd (and 4th) sacral nerves.

7.02 The thoracic duct:

A. lies anterior to the internal jugular vein.
B. lies posterior to the carotid sheath.
C. is anterior to the phrenic nerve at the level of the 7th cervical vertebra.
D. crosses anterior to the oesophagus at the T4–T5 level.
E. in the posterior mediastinum lies anterior to the posterior intercostal arteries.

7.03 The ureter:

A. is the immediate anterior relation of the transverse processes of the 3rd and 4th lumbar vertebrae.
B. in the female passes just above the lateral fornix of the vagina.
C. on the right side is an anterior relation of the duodenum.
D. lies anterior to the genitofemoral nerve.
E. in the pelvis, has lymphatics which drain to the internal and external iliac lymph nodes.

Answers overleaf

7.01 A, B, C, D, E.
An example of all true items just to remind the reader that all or none of the items in a question may be correct. The plexus at the side of the rectum (inferior hypogastric plexus) also receives sympathetic branches from the presacral nerve (superior hypogastric plexus).

7.02 B, C, E.
The thoracic duct is posterior to the internal jugular vein and crosses behind the oesophagus at the level of T4–T5.

7.03 B, D, E.
The ureter lies behind the peritoneum on the medial part of the psoas major. On the right side the ureter is usually posterior to the descending part of the duodenum.

7.04 The inguinal canal:

A. transmits the ilio-inguinal nerve in both sexes.
B. has the internal oblique muscle along the whole length of its anterior wall.
C. has the fascia transversalis and conjoint tendon along its posterior wall.
D. in the newborn, is more oblique than in the adult.
E. transmits the genital branch of the genitofemoral nerve in the female.

7.05 The spinal cord:

A. has a central canal containing cerebrospinal fluid.
B. is held in place by the denticulate ligaments.
C. is surrounded by two meningeal layers.
D. the blood supply is from three longitudinal arterial channels.
E. in the fetus at term usually terminates at the L3–L4 level.

7.06 In relation to the adult heart:

A. the pericardium consists of three layers.
B. the crista terminalis is inside the right atrium.
C. the trabeculated part of the right atrium has developed from the sinus venosus.
D. the interventricular septum is entirely muscular.
E. its oblique sinus is an immediate anterior relation of the oesophagus.

7.07 Which of the following are homologous structures in both sexes?

A. Labia minora — scrotum.
B. Ovarian ligament — gubernaculum of the testis.
C. Uterine tube — ductus deferens.
D. Duct of the epoophoron — duct of the epididymis.
E. Bartholin's glands — bulbo-urethral glands (Cowper's glands).

Answers overleaf

7.04 A, C, E.
The external oblique muscle is present along the whole length of the anterior wall, but the internal oblique muscle is only present laterally. In the newborn the canal is less oblique; it becomes more oblique with increasing age.

7.05 A, B, D, E.
The dura, arachnoid and pia mater clothe the spinal cord throughout its length.

7.06 A, B, E.
The trabeculated part of the definitive right atrium is formed from the right half of the original common atrium. The uppermost part of the interventricular septum is membranous and not muscular.

7.07 B, D, E.
The labia majora and scrotum are homologous. The uterine tube corresponds to the appendix of the testis and prostatic utricle (derived from the paramesonephric duct). The ductus deferens is derived from the mesonephric duct.

7.08 The ischiorectal fossa:

A. is bounded laterally by the obturator internus muscle.
B. is bounded medially by the rectum.
C. has a roof formed by the fascia of the levator ani muscle.
D. contains structures which have emerged from the pelvis through the obturator canal.
E. extends into the urogenital triangle.

7.09 In the fetal circulation:

A. the left umbilical vein drains into the ductus venosus.
B. the highest oxygen saturation is in the umbilical vein.
C. the right ventricular wall is thinner than the left ventricular wall.
D. the septum secundum grows down and becomes the limbus of the foramen ovale.
E. at birth, the umbilical arteries contract before the umbilical vein.

7.10 With regard to the pharyngeal arches and pharyngeal pouches in man.

A. The arches are masses of mesoderm covered with ectoderm and lined with entoderm.
B. The third arch is supplied by the glossopharyngeal nerve.
C. The first pouch gives rise to the Eustachian (auditory, pharyngotympanic) tube.
D. The second pouch swells to form the palatine tonsil.
E. The third pouch provides the primordia for the thymus.

Answers overleaf

7.08 A, C, E.
The medial wall of the ischiorectal fossa is formed by the inferior surface of the levator ani and its fascial covering. Below the levator ani, the external anal sphincter forms the medial wall. The ischiorectal fossa is a fat-filled space. The pudendal nerve and internal pudendal vessels enter the perineum through the lesser sciatic foramen, run in a fascial (pudendal, Alcock's) canal on the lateral wall of the fossa and give off inferior rectal branches. The fossa also contains the perineal branch of the 4th sacral nerve.

7.09 A, B, D, E.
The muscular wall of the right ventricle is thicker than the wall of the left ventricle, a condition which persists throughout fetal life but is rapidly reversed after birth.

7.10 A, B, C, D, E.
The questions involve basic facts which may not always be appreciated by obstetricians, but they should be aware of the principal derivatives of the pharyngeal arches and pouches.

7.11 The testes.

A. Venous drainage is to the vena cava on both sides.
B. The epididymis lies along its lateral part of its posterior border.
C. The right testicle hangs somewhat lower than the left.
D. Lymphatic drainage is to paraortic lymph nodes.
E. Contains interstitial cells which enlarge to become spermatogonia.

7.12 The mature human ovarian follicle:

A. is controlled throughout its development by luteinising hormone.
B. is surrounded by theca cells.
C. produces progesterone.
D. forms from one of a number of primary follicles which develop during each cycle.
E. ruptures at ovulation due to mechanical pressure of follicular fluid.

7.13 The breast:

A. is an exocrine gland.
B. is an apocrine gland.
C. develops at puberty before the onset of menstruation.
D. requires thyroxine for full development.
E. shows alveolar proliferation in man due to progesterone.

7.14 The vagina:

A. has a pH during reproductive life below 7.
B. is developed in its lower one-third from the Mullerian (paramesonephric) duct.
C. shows atrophy following reduced oestrogen stimulation.
D. in the presence of diabetes mellitus, it is predisposed to Trichomonas infection.
E. has an epithelium which thickens at puberty.

Answers overleaf

7.11 B, D.
On the left side the testicular vein opens into the left renal vein. The left testicle hangs about 1 cm lower than the right. The interstitial cells excrete testosterone.

7.12 D.
The ovarian follicle is not controlled throughout its development by LH; follicle-stimulating hormone is required initially. The ovum is surrounded by a single layer of follicular cells. The follicle itself does not produce hormones, the surrounding cells do. The precise mechanism of rupture of the follicle is unknown, but it is generally accepted that increased hydrostatic pressure within the follicle is not responsible for rupture at ovulation. It is probable that enzymes such as plasmin and collagenase are activated in the preovulatory period and digest the follicular wall. The increased amount of follicular fluid necroses the surface of the ovary and this gives way, but the actual mechanism of rupture of the follicular wall is enzymatic in nature.

7.13 A, B, C, E.
In females the breasts develop primarily under the control of oestrogens, which cause proliferation of the mammary ducts, and progesterone which results in the development of the lobules. During pregnancy, prolactin levels increase steadily until term, and with the high level of oestrogen and progesterone, full lobulo-alveolar development of the breast takes place. The actual size of the breast depends on genetic and nutritional factors.

7.14 A, C, E.
The lower third (or two-fifths) of the vagina is derived from the urogenital sinus epithelium. Diabetes mellitus is associated with Monilia infections **not** Trichomonas infections.

.15 In the early stages of the embryo:
- **A.** the zygote has the adult diploid number of chromosomes.
- **B.** the morula becomes implanted in the uterine wall after the loss of the zona pellucida.
- **C.** the extra-embryonic mesoderm contributes to the development of the chorion.
- **D.** the cloacal membrane gives rise to the allantois.
- **E.** the yolk sac becomes the vitelline duct in the body stalk.

.16 Non-myelinated nerve fibres are:
- **A.** associated with the sensation of pain.
- **B.** devoid of Schwann cell investment.
- **C.** characteristic of preganglionic neurons.
- **D.** devoid of nodes of Ranvier.
- **E.** confined to the grey matter of the spinal cord.

.17 The human placenta:
- **A.** produces pregnanediol.
- **B.** is haemochorial.
- **C.** has anastomoses between villous vessels.
- **D.** has syncytiotrophoblast as the major component of the trophoblast near term.
- **E.** is anchored to the myometrium by stem villi.

.18 In the normal human pelvis:
- **A.** the true pelvis is shallower during childhood prior to puberty.
- **B.** the sacrum is broader in the male.
- **C.** in the upright posture the pelvic surface of the symphysis faces upwards and backwards.
- **D.** in the sitting position the body rests on the ischial tuberosities.
- **E.** the ischial spines are more inverted in the male than in the female.

Answers overleaf

7.15 A, B, C, E.
The allantois is an endodermal diverticulum extending from the yolk sac into the body stalk. The cloaca is the common endodermal chamber into which the hindgut and allantois open.

7.16 A, D.
Nonmyelinated nerve fibres invaginate into a Schwann cell, and are characteristic of post-ganglionic fibres in the autonomic nervous system, and therefore not confined to the grey matter of the spinal cord.

7.17 B, C, D.
The placenta synthesises progesterone from cholesterol itself which is metabolised by the maternal liver and excreted in urine as pregnanediol. The decidua is not penetrated beyond the superficial part of the spongy layer.

7.18 A, C, D, E.
The sacrum is shorter and wider in the female and its upper part is straight.

.19 The human spermatozoon:

A. contain hyaluronidase in the acrosome.
B. contain adenosine triphosphate in the tail.
C. require the presence of follicle-stimulating hormone for normal development.
D. are concentrated in the seminal vesicles.
E. account for less than 10% of the volume of the ejaculate in man.

.20 In the embryo:

A. the heart is formed by the fusion of two tubes which invaginate the pericardium so that a dorsal mesentery is formed.
B. during development the inferior vena cava receives contributions from the right subcardinal vein.
C. the liver develops as a dorsal bud from the primitive gut.
D. the primitive midgut is extruded into the body stalk between the 6th and 12th week of intrauterine life.
E. the mammary glands are derived from the ectodermal germ layer.

Answers overleaf

7.19 A, B, C, E.
The seminal vesicles secrete an alkaline, yellow, viscid fluid which forms much of the volume of the ejaculated sperm.

7.20 A, B, D, E.
The hepatic primordium (bud or early rudiment) is a median thickening of the endoderm in contact with the septum transversum.

8. ENDOCRINOLOGY AND GENETICS

8.01 Luteinising hormone is:
A. a glycoprotein.
B. comprised of two subunits.
C. released intermittently.
D. increased in maternal blood throughout pregnancy.
E. bound to plasma proteins.

8.02 Deficient adrenal function causes:
A. hypotension.
B. peripheral vasodilation.
C. oedema.
D. hyperglycaemia.
E. acidosis.

8.03 Thyroxine:
A. stimulates cell metabolism.
B. is excreted in the urine.
C. decreases fat utilisation.
D. is bound to a globulin in the circulation.
E. is produced from tyrosine and inorganic iodine.

8.04 Ovulation in the human is associated with:
A. a surge of luteinising hormone.
B. a fall in serum follicle-stimulating hormone.
C. increased viscosity of cervical mucus.
D. increased vascularity of theca interna.
E. absence of spinnbarkeit formation.

Answers overleaf

8.01 A, B, C.
Luteinising hormone is not increased in pregnancy, although high levels of HCG are present during pregnancy. There is a considerable overlap in the amino acid sequence of HCG and the alpha-subunit of LH. Indeed, HCG can only be distinguished from LH by antisera raised against the beta-subunit of HCG. LH is not bound to plasma proteins, it exists in a free state.

8.02 A, B, E.
The clinical features of acute adrenal insufficiency are profound shock, muscular weakness, hypotension, oligurea, urea retention, rise in plasma [K^+], initial fever and subsequent hypothermia, vomiting and dehydration. Plasma [Na^+] falls, mainly due to the altered distribution of Na^+ and water between cells and extracellular fluid. Chronic insufficiency is associated with muscular weakness, pigmentation of skin, loss of weight, and dehydration, hypotension, anorexia, nausea, vomiting and diarrhoea, mental confusion, symptoms of hypoglycaemia, decreased growth of body hair, decreased ability to withstand trauma, infection, haemorrhage and other stress factors.

8.03 A, B, D, E.
All tissue metabolism is influenced by thyroid hormones. Thyroxine increases free fatty acid production and therefore utilisation.

8.04 A, D.
There is a modest rise of FSH at ovulation. The cervical mucus is increased in quantity, and there is development of spinnbarkeit.

.05 The children of a father heterozygous for a given autosomal gene:

A. have a 1 in 4 chance of being a heterozygote if the mother is also a heterozygote.
B. have a 1 in 4 chance of being a heterozygote if the mother does not carry the gene.
C. have a 1 in 2 chance of being a heterozygote if the mother is homozygous for the gene.
D. have a 1 in 4 chance of being a homozygote if the mother is a heterozygote.
E. have a 1 in 4 chance of not carrying the gene if the mother is a heterozygote.

.06 Adrenocorticotrophic hormone (ACTH):

A. is produced by nerve cells in the hypothalamus.
B. has a greater effect on aldosterone secretion than on cortisol secretion.
C. output is decreased by a fall in the circulating cortisol level.
D. output is controlled by a releasing factor from the hypothalamus.
E. is a polypeptide.

.07 Conception is less likely to occur:

A. when sexual intercourse is restricted to the 7th–21st days of a 28-day menstrual cycle.
B. in fertile women aged 40–44 than in those aged 20–24.
C. if the male partner has bilateral cryptorchism.
D. in untreated diabetes mellitus.
E. if clomiphene citrate is given from the 6th to the 10th day of a 28-day menstrual cycle.

.08 In Klinefelter's syndrome there is:

A. a male phenotype.
B. more than one X chromosome.
C. a lower incidence of mental retardation.
D. a raised urinary excretion of pituitary gonadotrophin.
E. gonadal dysgenesis.

Answers overleaf

8.05 C, D, E.
The chances for A are 2 out of 4 and for B, 1 out of 2.

8.06 D, E.
ACTH is produced from the basophil cells of the anterior pituitary gland. It controls the growth and biological activity of the adrenal cortex, which secretes the principal glucocorticoid cortisol. Its secretion is subject to influences from the circadian rhythm, negative cortisol feedback and response to stress.

8.07 B, C, D.
In a 28-day menstrual cycle, the fertile period is likely to be the 14th day plus or minus 3 or 4 days. Clomiphene citrate stimulates ovulation whether given on the 2nd–6th or 6th–10th days inclusive of the menstrual cycle.

8.08 A, B, D, E.
Mental retardation is a recognised feature of Klinefelter's syndrome.

8.09 Human cytogenetics.

A. Trisomic cells contain 3 pairs of a particular chromosome.
B. Diploid cells contain homologous pairs of chromosomes.
C. Chromosome homologues exchange portions of chromatids during mitosis.
D. Haploid cells contain 23 chromosomes.
E. Aneuploid cells contain an abnormal number of chromosomes.

8.10 Cortisol:

A. is catabolised in the liver.
B. blood levels increase following stress.
C. enhances protein synthesis.
D. enhances the effects of antigen–antibody reactions.
E. reduces the normal blood pressure.

8.11 Which of the following genetic disorders are inherited as X-linked recessives?

A. Neurofibromatosis (Von Recklinghausen's disease).
B. Haemophilia A.
C. Phenylketonuria.
D. Duchenne muscular dystrophy.
E. Glucose-6-phosphate dehydrogenase deficiency.

8.12 Down's syndrome (mongolism):

A. has an increased incidence of chronic myeloid leukaemia.
B. has an increased incidence with advancing maternal age.
C. can be caused by a paternal 14/21 translocation.
D. of the G21 trisomy type is associated with a normal maternal chromosomal pattern.
E. is characterised by patent ductus arteriosus.

Answers overleaf

8.09 B, D, E.
There are 3 chromosomes in a trisomic cell. Trisomy is the presence of one chromosome additional to the normal diploid set (i.e. 47 in man). Portions of chromatids are exchanged during meiosis.

8.10 A, B, C.
Cortisol in general inhibits inflammatory and allergic reactions. It has no direct effect on blood pressure.

8.11 B, D, E.
Neurofibromatosis is a dominant condition and phenylketonuria is an autosomal recessive conditon.

8.12 A, B, C, D.
The condition is characterised by endocardial cushion defects, not patent ductus arteriosus.

8.13 Congenital abnormalities.

A. Mongol children born to mothers under the age of 25 years may show chromosome abnormalities of the trisomy type.
B. Congenital pyloric stenosis occurs more frequently in relatives of affected infants than in the general population.
C. All daughters of a female carrier of red–green colour blindness are themselves carriers.
D. In anencephaly, alpha-fetoprotein (AFP) levels in amnoitic fluid are lower than normal.
E. Sickle cell disease is sex linked.

8.14 Which of the following relatives of a male child with haemophilia A are also at risk of having the same disorder of blood clotting?

A. His father.
B. His son.
C. Father's brother.
D. Mother's brother.
E. His brother.

8.15 The pituitary gland:

A. anterior lobe develops from the alimentary tract.
B. posterior lobe is largely influenced by hormones passing down blood vessels in the pituitary stalk.
C. anterior lobe has a direct neuroregulatory mechanism.
D. secretes releasing factors.
E. posterior lobe is developed from the brain.

8.16 Familial hypophosphataemia is characterised by:

A. impaired renal tubular function.
B. inheritance by an autosomal recessive gene.
C. impaired calcium absorption from the bowel.
D. decreased renal excretion of phosphate.
E. a low serum phosphorus level.

Answers overleaf

8.13 A, B.
The risk of being a carrier in item C is 1 out of 2, so not all daughters will be affected. The amniotic AFP levels are raised when anencephaly is present. Sickle cell disease is an autosomal recessive condition.

8.14 D, E.
The condition is X-linked, not Y-linked.

8.15 A, E.
The anterior lobe is activated through the hypophyseal portal venous system. The posterior lobe is a secretory and storage unit comprising neural tissue, and the release of vasopressin or antidiuretic hormone (ADH) and oxytocin is controlled by neurogenic stimuli; there is no intercommunicating system of portal vessels. There are no releasing factors produced.

8.16 A, C, E.
This is a rare inherited disorder which is a sex-linked dominant characteristic, the abnormal allele being on the X chromosome and males being more severely affected. The reabsorption of filtered phosphate is markedly impaired and the plasma phosphate is reduced.

.17 The hypothalamus:

A. forms part of the midbrain.
B. is closely related to the optic tract.
C. exerts specific actions by means of releasing factors.
D. is influenced by endocrine gland secretions.
E. has nerve connections with the anterior lobe of the pituitary gland.

.18 Iodine:

A. uptake by the thyroid gland is by passive diffusion.
B. uptake by the thyroid is influenced by the posterior pituitary gland.
C. ingestion is necessary for normal thyroid function.
D. requirements are increased in adolescence.
E. requirements are increased during lactation.

3.19 Which of the following substances when administered to a normal non-pregnant individual will increase the rate of insulin secretion?

A. Glucagon.
B. Glucose.
C. Adrenaline.
D. Noradrenaline.
E. Oestrogens.

3.20 Oxytocin:

A. is essential for the maintenance of pregnancy.
B. stimulates the myoepithelial cells of the lactating breast.
C. is synthesised mainly in the paraventricular nucleus.
D. is active in the male.
E. secretion rate is increased by stress.

Answers overleaf

8.17 B, C, D.
The hypothalamus is in an area of the forebrain, situated above the pituitary gland and forming the anteroinferior wall and floor of the third ventricle. It is bordered laterally by the optic tracts and cerebral peduncles and anteriorly by the optic chiasma. The connection from the hypothalamus to the anterior lobe of the pituitary gland is through the hyperphyseal portal venous system.

8.18 C, D, E.
Iodine is trapped and concentrated within the thyroid gland. It is converted to iodide and absorbed, and the iodide actively transported from the circulation to the colloid. TSH influences thyroid functions and it comes from the anterior pituitary and affects iodide binding.

8.19 A, B, E.
Adrenaline and noradrenaline would, in general, reduce insulin secretion but obviously the effect is dose dependent.

8.20 B, C.
Oxytocin is released physiologically in two situations, namely, in the final stages of labour and in the puerperium in response to sucking.

9. BIOCHEMISTRY

9.01 Vitamin A:

A. is water soluble.
B. requires bile for its absorption.
C. excess leads to xerophthalmia.
D. deficiency leads to night blindness.
E. is stored in the liver.

9.02 Urea:

A. is formed from amino acids.
B. is the main non-protein form of nitrogen in serum.
C. contributes about 80% of plasma non-protein nitrogen.
D. is synthesised in the liver.
E. does not enter red blood cells.

9.03 Hypokalaemia occurs in association with:

A. renal tubular acidosis.
B. hyperparathyroidism.
C. hormone-secreting tumours of the bronchus.
D. atrophy of the adrenal cortex.
E. pituitary tumour causing Cushing's syndrome.

9.04 Plasma enzyme levels.

A. Lipase rises in acute pancreatitis.
B. Amylase falls in acute pancreatitis.
C. Lactic dehydrogenase rises in leukaemia.
D. Serum transaminase falls in myocardial infarction.
E. Alkaline phosphatase rises in hyperparathyroidism.

Answers overleaf

9.01 D, E.
Vitamin A is fat soluble and is handled by the gastrointestinal system in the same manner as dietary fat. Once absorbed, the lipid-soluble vitamins are transported to the liver and either stored in the liver (A, D, K) or in adipose tissue (E) for varying periods of time. The full syndrome of vitamin A deficiency includes xeroderma, xerophthalmia, ketomalacia, severe growth retardation (including that of the nervous system), glandular degeneration and sterility.

9.02 A, B, D, E.
The amount of non-protein nitrogen in the serum or blood is 15–35 mg/dl (10.7–25 nmol/l) and the urea nitrogen is 8–20 mg/dl (2.86–7.14 nmol/l).

9.03 A, C, E.
Hyperparathyroidism is associated with hypercalcaemia. Atrophy of the adrenal cortex is associated with hyperkalaemia.

9.04 A, C, E.
The serum amylase rises in acute pancreatitis. There is a rapid and striking rise in serum transaminase levels following myocardial infarction.

9.05 Iron-binding capacity of the serum is:
- **A.** a measure of the transferrin content.
- **B.** normally 250–400 μg/dl (45–70 μmol/l).
- **C.** normally about 90% saturated.
- **D.** higher in women than in men.
- **E.** raised in pregnancy.

9.06 Vitamin K:
- **A.** is present in green vegetables.
- **B.** is water soluble.
- **C.** is synthesised by bacteria.
- **D.** is stored in large quantities in the liver.
- **E.** deficiency causes hypoprothrombinaemia.

9.07 Haemopoietic activity in the bone marrow is typically increased:
- **A.** following injections of cyanocobalamin (vitamin B_{12}) into a healthy individual on a normal diet.
- **B.** following haemorrhage.
- **C.** when the reticulocyte count is high in the peripheral blood.
- **D.** in a patient suffering from haemolytic anaemia.
- **E.** at high altitude.

9.08 Which of the following enzymes can break adrenaline (epinephrine)?
- **A.** Catechol-O-methyl transferase.
- **B.** Monoamine oxidase.
- **C.** Serum aspartate transaminase.
- **D.** Pseudocholinesterase.
- **E.** Dopamine-β-hydroxylase.

Answers overleaf

9.05 A, B, E.
The plasma is normally about 30% saturated with iron. There is no difference in iron-binding capacity between men and women.

9.06 A, C, E.
Vitamin K is fat soluble. Although vitamin K accumulates initially in the liver, its hepatic concentration declines rapidly.

9.07 B, C, D, E.
Vitamin B_{12} only exerts its effect in the presence of a deficiency.

9.08 A, B.
Adrenaline is primarily synthesised and stored in the adrenal medulla and acts through the circulation on distant organs. Most of the hormone is metabolised in tissues by a series of methylations of the phenolic groups or oxidations on the amine side-chains. The main enzymes involved are monoamine oxidase for oxidation reactions and catechol-O-methyl transferase (COMT) for catalysis of the methylations. A given enzyme catalyses very few reactions (frequently only one). Enzyme names have two parts: the first names the substrate or substrates, the second, ending in -ase, indicates the type of reaction catalysed.

9.09 Characteristics of renin are that:
- **A.** it is a lipid.
- **B.** its activity depends on the presence of a specific plasma protein.
- **C.** it is produced in the liver.
- **D.** it acts on a globulin substrate to form angiotensin I.
- **E.** its concentration in the blood is raised in normal pregnancy.

9.10 The condition known as phenylketonuria:
- **A.** can be diagnosed soon after birth.
- **B.** has a defective phenylalanine hydroxylase enzyme.
- **C.** has a high blood tyrosine level.
- **D.** is associated with the presence of phenylpyruvic acid in the urine.
- **E.** is associated with a raised blood phenylalanine level.

9.11 With regard to deoxyribonucleic (DNA) acids.
- **A.** *Esch. coli* contains double-stranded DNA.
- **B.** Smallpox virus is an example of a DNA virus.
- **C.** Polioviruses are examples of DNA viruses.
- **D.** The influenza viruses are DNA viruses.
- **E.** Herpes simplex virus is an example of a DNA virus.

9.12 Cholesterol:
- **A.** is a major constituent of fungi.
- **B.** is synthesised from acetyl-co-enzyme A.
- **C.** is a constituent of many lipoproteins.
- **D.** is a component of mucopolysaccharides.
- **E.** is required for the synthesis of bile acids in the liver.

Answers overleaf

9.09 B, D, E.
Renin is an enzyme produced in the kidney acting on an alpha-2-globulin substrate to form an inactive decapeptide (angiotensin I). This is converted by another enzyme to angiotensin II which increases blood pressure.

9.10 A, B, D, E.
The condition is associated with the absence of the hepatic enzyme which normally converts any dietary phenylalanine not utilised into tyrosine, therefore the blood tyrosine levels will be low.

9.11 A, B, E.
Plant viruses all contain RNA, whereas nearly all bacteriophages contain DNA. Of the animal viruses affecting man, some contain DNA and some contain RNA. The polioviruses contain RNA, as do the influenza viruses.

9.12 B, C, E.
The walls of fungi contain glucan, polysaccharides and proteins. Lipids are present in the walls of some yeasts. Cholesterol is a lipid.

9.13 Calcitonin:

A. is a phospholipid.
B. inhibits the synthesis of dihydrocholecalciferol.
C. increases calcium excretion.
D. inhibits the action of osteoclasts.
E. originated from the C cells of the thyroid.

9.14 Which of the following factors affect acid–base balance?

A. Severe exercise.
B. Hyperventilation.
C. High-protein diet.
D. Iron deficiency anaemia.
E. Diabetes insipidus.

9.15 Lipoproteins contain:

A. cholesterol.
B. ergosterol.
C. triglycerides.
D. phospholipids.
E. apoproteins.

9.16 Water balance.

A. The obligatory water losses vary with diet.
B. The oxidation of 1 g of protein yields more water than the oxidation of 1 g of fat.
C. The minimum obligatory daily urine output is over 1 litre.
D. In health the total body water varies less than 1% of the body weight per day.
E. The regulatory system is located in the hypothalamus.

Answers overleaf

9.13 B, C, D, E.
Calcitonin is a peptide containing 32 amino acids.

9.14 A, B, C.
There is no way in which anaemia or diabetes insipidus should affect acid–base balance.

9.15 A, C, D, E.
Ergosterol occurs in plants and yeast. It is important as a precursor of vitamin D.

9.16 A, D, E.
The minimum obligatory daily urine volume is 700–750 ml, depending to some extent on the diet. The oxidation of 1 g each of starch, protein and fat yields 0.6, 0.4 and 1.07 g of water, respectively. The amount of metabolic water is quite small relative to that ingested in food or drink.

9.17 Which of the following iron compounds are correctly paired with their function in health?

A. Myoglobin — oxygen storage.
B. Transferrin — iron transport.
C. Ferritin — iron transport.
D. Cytochrome — oxidation.
E. Haemosiderin — iron storage.

9.18 Which of the following minerals and trace elements are correctly paired with their functions?

A. Magnesium — enzyme co-factor.
B. Copper — oxidase enzymes.
C. Chromium — nerve and muscle function.
D. Zinc — enzyme co-factor.
E. Phosphorus — metabolic intermediaries.

9.19 Histamine:

A. is derived from histadine.
B. is an essential amino acid.
C. is present in the mast cells of tissues.
D. is present in platelets.
E. stimulates the secretion of hydrochloric acid by the stomach.

9.20 Blood clotting factors.

A. Fibrinogen is a soluble plasma protein.
B. Prothrombin is synthesised in the liver.
C. Plasmin is capable of digesting fibrin.
D. Prothrombin activator is only formed as a result of tissue damage.
E. The conversion of Factor X to its active form takes place within a few seconds.

Answers overleaf

9.17 A, B, D, E.
Ferritin in the reticuloendothelial system provides an available storage form for iron.

9.18 A, B, D, E.
Chromium is thought to play some functional role in the regulation of glucose metabolism. There have been suggestions that it is important in the metabolism of proteins and lipids, particularly cholesterol.

9.19 A, C, D, E.
Histamine is not an essential amino acid. (See question 3.15 and its answer for the list of essential amino acids.)

9.20 A, B, C.
Prothrombin activator (also called thromboplastin) is formed in two ways: one as the result of tissue damage, and the other by activation of an intrinsic system consisting entirely of blood constituents. The statement in **E** is incorrect as once the active form of Factor X (i.e. Xa) is formed, clotting takes place in seconds; the preceding stages take longer.

10. PHYSIOLOGY

10.01 The surfactant material lining the lung alveoli:

A. increases the surface tension of the alveolar fluid.
B. increases the compliance of the lungs.
C. consists of molecules which are partly water soluble and partly fat soluble.
D. is decreased when pulmonary blood flow is interrupted.
E. is present in the amnoitic fluid.

10.02 The carotid bodies:

A. have, for their size, a richer blood supply than that of brain tissue.
B. respond to alterations in blood pressure.
C. are stimulated by a rise in blood hydrogen ion concentration.
D. are stimulated by a fall in blood flow.
E. receive afferent fibres from the respiratory centre.

10.03 Pancreatic juice:

A. is secreted from the islets of Langerhans.
B. contains proteolytic enzymes.
C. enzyme secretion is stimulated by pancreozymin.
D. bicarbonate secretion is stimulated by enterokinase.
E. contains an inhibitor of trypsin.

10.04 During pregnancy:

A. venous tone is reduced.
B. the output of maternal parathormone is elevated.
C. there is an increase in the circulating fibrinogen level.
D. there is a rise in cardiac output.
E. the renal threshold for glucose rises.

Answers overleaf

10.01 B, C, D, E.
Surfactant reduces the surface tension of the alveolar fluid.

10.02 A, C, D.
The carotid and aortic bodies are 'chemoreceptors'. The sensory innervation of the carotid body is from glossopharyngeal and vagus nerves.

10.03 B, C, E.
The islets of Langerhans secrete glucagon from the alpha-cells and insulin from the beta-cells. Enterokinase is an enzyme secreted by the duodenal mucosa and converts trypsinogen to trypsin.

10.04 A, B, C, D.
The renal threshold for glucose is lowered due to the fact that renal reabsorption of glucose is less effective in pregnancy.

.05 Renal function.

A. The kidneys receive 10–15% of the cardiac output.
B. The average glomerular filtration rate in the normal adult male is 120–130 ml/min.
C. The glomerular filtration rate can be determined by the inulin clearance test.
D. The kidneys regulate blood volume.
E. The kidneys actively reabsorb glucose in the proximal tubules.

.06 The oxyhaemoglobin dissociation curve:

A. when displaced to the left, means greater avidity of Hb for O_2.
B. is displaced to the left by a raised temperature.
C. is unaffected by pH.
D. expresses the oxygen saturation of haemoglobin as a function of $P\text{O}_2$.
E. is displaced to the right at high altitude.

.07 In arterial blood:

A. 18–20 ml/dl of oxygen is in combination with haemoglobin.
B. there is a carbon dioxide tension of 38–42 mmHg.
C. a reduced $P\text{CO}_2$ due to hyperventilation occurs in normal pregnancy.
D. carbon dioxide is carried mostly by bicarbonate.
E. carbon dioxide is carried in reduced amounts at low atmospheric pressure.

.08 Fetal haemoglobin (HbF):

A. is not formed before 10 weeks.
B. is less resistant than adult haemoglobin to denaturation by alkali.
C. constitutes 80–90% of the haemoglobin of the fetus at term.
D. is less than 5% 8 weeks after birth.
E. is found in adult patients with sickle cell anaemia.

Answers overleaf

10.05 B, C, E.
The kidneys receive 20–25% of the cardiac output. They excrete urine, and many homoeostatic regulatory mechanisms minimise or prevent changes in the extracellular fluid by exchanging the amount of water and various solutes in the urine. They do not regulate blood volume.

10.06 A, D, E.
It is displaced to the right by a raised temperature. Physiological shifts of the dissociation curve are *related* to changes in hydrion, CO_2 2,3-diphosphoglycerate (2,3-DPG) and temperature.

10.07 A, B, C, D, E.
All basic facts.

10.08 A, C.
Haemoglobin first appears in the fetal circulation at about the 20th week, when the bone marrow begins to function. Adult haemoglobin (HbA) is rapidly denatured by alkali, but fetal haemoglobin (HbF) is more resistant and forms the basis of the Kleihauer test. HbF is largely replaced by HbA in the first year of life. Sickle cell disease and sickle cell trait are related to haemoglobin S.

0.09 During 'isometric' ventricular contraction:
- **A.** pressure is rising steadily in the aorta.
- **B.** the valves of the ventricle are closed.
- **C.** blood flow to ventricular muscle falls.
- **D.** there is little muscle shortening.
- **E.** intraventricular pressure falls.

0.10 When standing, the venous pressure:
- **A.** in the jugular vein is subatmospheric.
- **B.** in the foot is about 100 mmHg.
- **C.** in the thorax decreases when the subject inspires.
- **D.** increases in pressure from the venules to the larger veins.
- **E.** in the superior vena cava is between 4 and 6 mmHg.

0.11 Arterioles:
- **A.** have a thicker wall in relation to the lumen than other blood vessels.
- **B.** play a major role in the regulation of arterial blood pressure.
- **C.** contain more elastic tissue relative to their size than does the aorta.
- **D.** play a major role in regulating local blood flow.
- **E.** may connect directly with venules.

0.12 During normal pregnancy which of the following are increased?
- **A.** Respiratory rate.
- **B.** Tidal volume.
- **C.** Inspiratory capacity.
- **D.** Expiratory reserve volume.
- **E.** Alveolar ventilation.

Answers overleaf

10.09 B, C, D.
The pressure in the aorta is steady during isometric (isovolumetric) contraction and rises steadily in the ventricular ejection phase. During this phase the intraventricular pressure rises.

10.10 A, B, C, E.
The pressure in the venules is 12–18 mmHg and it falls steadily in the larger veins to about 5.5 mmHg in the great veins outside the thorax.

10.11 A, B, D, E.
The arterioles contain less elastic tissue but much more smooth muscle than the aorta and larger arteries.

10.12 B, C, E.
The respiratory rate does not increase in pregnancy, and the expiratory reserve volume falls.

0.13 Stimulation of the respiratory centres by carbon dioxide:
A. is entirely due to its effect on the pH of the blood.
B. leads to an increased respiratory rate without increased ventilation.
C. is reduced by morphine.
D. is increased by aminophylline.
E. is increased by progesterone.

0.14 Active erythropoietic tissue:
A. first appears in the bone marrow during the last 3 months of intrauterine life.
B. occupies the whole bone marrow at birth.
C. is replaced by fat in the long bones of the healthy adult.
D. is not found in the vertebrae of adults.
E. is present in the flat bones of the healthy adult.

0.15 Cardiac output:
A. is usually expressed as the combined output per minute of both ventricles.
B. need not increase when the heart rate rises.
C. rises when the subject changes from the standing to the lying down position.
D. is unaffected by sleep.
E. is reduced when eating a meal.

0.16 Pancreatic secretions:
A. increase the conversion of lactose to glucose.
B. increase fat absorption.
C. decrease liver glycogen.
D. decrease sucrose absorption.
E. include amylase.

Answers overleaf

10.13 C, D, E.
Various stimuli affect the respiratory centre. There is chemical control by CO_2 (via CSF hydrogen ion concentration), O_2 and H^+ via the carotid and aortic bodies, as well as non-chemical control by afferents from proprioreceptors, afferents for sneezing, coughing, swallowing, yawning, vagal afferents from inflation and deflation receptors, and afferents from the baroreceptors. The respiratory rate and ventilation are increased.

10.14 B, C, E.
Haemopoiesis in the fetal bone marrow begins at about week 16 and increases progressively. In the adult, red marrow, which contains numerous blood cells of all kinds and their precursors, persists mainly in the vertebrae, sternum, ribs and bones of the skull and pelvis.

10.15 B, C, D.
The cardiac output is the amount of blood pumped out of each ventricle per unit time, usually per minute. In general there is about a 30% increase in cardiac output when eating a meal.

10.16 B, C, E.
This question could be considered ambiguous because there is no indication if both endocrine and exocrine secretions are to be considered. If both then **C** is true, if only exocrine substances, **C** would be false. This illustrates the care required to obtain good MCQs. The answer to **C** will vary according to your interpretation of pancreatic secretions. Lactose is digested in the small intestine by secretions of Brunner's glands of the duodenum and glands of Lieberkühn. It has no effect on sucrose absorption.

10.17 Systolic blood pressure:

A. in the circulation is directly related to the peripheral resistance.
B. is directly related to cardiac output.
C. is dependent on the baroreceptors.
D. is independent of the chemoreceptors.
E. is unaffected by gravity.

10.18 Cardiac muscle:

A. contraction depends upon an interaction between actin and myosin filaments.
B. contraction is enhanced when the serum potassium rises above normal.
C. contraction is dependent upon the presence of calcium ions.
D. has the ability to retract.
E. has an inherent rhythmicity.

10.19 The fetal circulation.

A. The ductus venosus carries blood to the inferior vena cava from the umbilical artery.
B. The ductus arteriosus carries blood from the pulmonary artery to the aorta.
C. The foramen ovale permits blood to pass from the right to the left ventricle.
D. The inferior vena cava contains oxygenated blood.
E. The ductus arteriosus is contractile.

10.20 In a normal electrocardiogram:

A. the QRS complex is of variable amplitude.
B. the T wave represents slow ventricular depolarisation.
C. the T wave is asymmetrical.
D. the ascending segment of the T wave is longer than the descending.
E. the QRS complex represents rapid ventricular repolarisation.

Answers overleaf

10.17 C, D.
The main factors determining the systolic pressure are the diastolic pressure, the stroke volume of the heart and the aortic elasticity. Diastolic pressure depends on the systolic pressure, the systemic resistance and heart rate. Both systolic and diastolic pressures are influenced by the blood volume. The barorecepors constitute a reflex feedback mechanism that operates to stabilise the blood pressure and heart rate. Blood pressure is affected by gravity and position.

10.18 A, C, E.
As in other excitable tissues, changes in the external potassium concentration affect the resting membrane potential of cardiac muscle. Hyperkalaemia is a very dangerous and potentially lethal condition because of its effect on the heart and the contractions are reduced or paralysed. Uterine muscle is the only one with the property of retraction.

10.19 B, D, E.
The ductus venosus carries blood from the umbilical vein. The foramen ovale permits blood to pass from the right atrium to the left atrium.

10.20 A, C, D.
QRS represents the stage of ventricular depolarisation. The ST and T waves represent the stage of repolarisation.

11. PATHOLOGY AND IMMUNOLOGY

11.01 In the presence of a phaeochromocytoma:

A. there may be hypertension.
B. there is an increased urinary excretion of catecholamines.
C. there is hypoglycaemia.
D. the basal metabolic rate is increased.
E. aldosterone production increases.

11.02 Carcinoma 'in situ' of the uterine cervix:

A. arises most commonly at the squamocolumnar junction.
B. has a peak age incidence of 50–55 years.
C. becomes invasive in 70–80% of cases.
D. involves the mucous glands of the endocervix.
E. is predominantly squamous in type.

11.03 Immunoglobulins.

A. The basic immunoglobulin molecule consists of 4 peptide chains.
B. Immunoglobulin G (IgG) can cross the placenta.
C. Immunoglobulin A (IgA) is able to fix complement by itself.
D. Immunoglobulin M (IgM) is a cryoglobulin.
E. Immunoglobulin M in the fetus is derived from the mother by placental transfer.

Answers overleaf

11.01 A, B, D.
Phaeochromocytoma usually produces adrenaline and noradrenaline to produce systemic hypertension, which is characteristically paroxysmal. If the tumour secretes adrenaline only, there may also be hyperglycaemia (noradrenaline does not have this effect). The tumour arises in the adrenal medulla or elsewhere where chromaffin tissue exists.

11.02 A, D, E.
The peak age incidence for carcinoma of the cervix is at 50–55; but, in general, it is accepted that the peak for CIN III is about 10 years earlier. Only about a third of in situ lesions progress to invasive disease.

11.03 A, B, D.
Immunoglobulin G fixes complement. Immunoglobulin A is the major immunoglobulin of the external secretions (interstitial fluids, saliva, bronchial excretions etc.). It does not fix complement except in the presence of lysozyme or, in polymerised form, via an alternative pathway. Immunoglobulin M does not cross the placenta in man, but may do so in certain species.

11.04 Rhesus isoimmunisation.

A. It is reduced if there is parenteral ABO incompatibility.

B. It can usually be prevented by giving anti-D globulin after delivery.

C. The Kleihauer (acid-elution) test can demonstrate fetal red cells in the maternal blood.

D. The umbilical cord haemoglobin level at birth reflects the severity of the haemolytic process.

E. There is a high titre of maternal IgM in the cord blood.

11.05 A transfusion reaction is likely to follow administration of:

A. group A blood to a group B person.

B. group O blood to a group AB person.

C. group A blood to a group O person.

D. group A blood to a group AB person.

E. group B blood to a group A person.

11.06 Lymphocytes.

A. Bursa-derived lymphocytes (B-cells) may develop into plasma cells.

B. B-cells produce specific immunoglobulin (IgG).

C. B-cells play a major role as antigen reactive cells.

D. B-cells are independent of thymus-derived lymphocytes (T-cells) in their actions.

E. T-cells are cytotoxic.

Answers overleaf

11.04 A, B, C, D.
The level of IgM is very low in the umbilical cord.

11.05 A, C, E.
Basic facts. There will be no reaction in the instances quoted in items **B** and **D**.

11.06 A, B, E.
T-lymphocytes (T-cells) not B-cells play a major role as antigen reactive cells and effector cells in cell mediated immunity, and cooperate with B-lymphocytes in antibody production (humoral immunity).

11.07 Granulation tissue:

A. is a feature of wound healing.
B. is present in the wall of an abscess.
C. forms the capsule of a uterine fibroid.
D. leads to scar tissue formation.
E. is a feature of amyloidosis.

11.08 In which of the following paired conditions is the second condition a characteristic sequel of the first?

A. Mastoiditis — meningitis.
B. Bronchiectasis — cerebral abscess.
C. Mumps — ovarian inflammation.
D. Bacillary dysentery — liver abscess.
E. Empyema of gall bladder — empyema of pleura.

11.09 Which of the following substances may be produced by neoplasms?

A. Dexamethasone.
B. 5-hydroxy-tryptamine.
C. Gonadotrophin.
D. Testosterone.
E. Insulin.

11.10 An abnormal number of red blood cells is found in the urine in:

A. *Schistosoma haematobium* infection.
B. sickle cell anaemia.
C. an incompatible blood transfusion.
D. pregnancy.
E. the presence of a renal adenocarcinoma.

Answers overleaf

11.07 A, B, D.
There is a false capsule around leiomyoma of the uterus, but it does not consist of granulation tissue. The salient features of amyloidosis is the extracellular deposition of an eosinophilic hyaline material.

11.08 A, B, C.
Bacillary dysentery is associated with intestinal ulceration, not abscess formation. Empyema is a collection of pus in a cavity and, in the case of empyema of the gall bladder, it follows acute cholecystitis.

11.09 B, C, D, E.
Dexamethasone is a drug used in corticosteroid therapy.

11.10 A, B, C, E.
An abnormal number of red blood cells is not generally present in uncomplicated pregnancies.

1.11 Chemical mediators concerned in the production of an inflammatory response include which of the following?

A. 5-Hydroxytryptamine.
B. Corticosteroids.
C. Globulin permeability factor.
D. Bradykinin.
E. Antihistamine.

1.12 Benign cystic teratomata (dermoid cyst) of the ovary:

A. have no mesodermal derivative.
B. frequently become malignant.
C. are bilateral in 25% of cases.
D. are sometimes detected by x-rays.
E. characteristically cause amenorrhoea.

1.13 Ulceration of the small bowel mucosa is characteristic of which of the following diseases?

A. Coeliac disease.
B. Amoebic dysentery.
C. Tuberculous enteritis.
D. Regional ileitis.
E. Typhoid fever.

1.14 Antibody formation.

A. This occurs in bursa-derived lymphocytes (B-cells).
B. It requires the co-operation of thymus-derived lymphocytes (T-cells).
C. It requires complement.
D. It involves conversion of pre-existing non-specific immunoglobulin (IgG)
E. Antigen–antibody reactions are characteristically suppressed by adrenocorticotrophic hormone.

Answers overleaf

11.11 A, C, D.
Whereas corticosteroids and antihistamines could be considered as chemical mediators in certain circumstances, they are not concerned in the production of an inflammatory response.

11.12 C, D.
Cystic adult teratomata (dermoids) are composed of all three germinal layers, although epithelial structures predominate. Only about 2% of cystic teratomata are complicated by malignancy. They exert no influence on the menstrual/ovarian cycle.

11.13 C, D, E.
Coeliac disease affects the small intestine, particularly the duodenum and jejunum. The characteristic mucosal change is 'subtotal villous atrophy'. It is essentially a malabsorption syndrome. Amoebic dysentery predominantly affects the colon, and therefore this would be considered a false answer although ulceration does occur.

11.14 A, B, E.
Complement is activated by many antigen–antibody reactions but is not required for antibody formation. IgG is the major immunoglobulin in the serum of man (800–1600 mg/dl). The primary function of an antibody is to combine with an antigen, which may alone be enough to neutralise, for example, toxins or some viruses. This action can be further increased by the ability of many antibodies to activate complement.

1.15 Anaemia in pregnancy may result from:
- **A.** folic acid deficiency.
- **B.** vitamin D deficiency.
- **C.** iron deficiency.
- **D.** chronic pyelonephritis.
- **E.** multiple pregnancy.

1.16 Pulmonary hypertension is a recognised complication of:
- **A.** thromboembolic disease.
- **B.** polycythaemia rubra vera.
- **C.** life at high altitude.
- **D.** choriocarcinoma.
- **E.** patent ductus arteriosus.

1.17 Which of the following haemoglobins are normally found in the human red blood cell at some stage of life?
- **A.** Haemoglobin A.
- **B.** Haemoglobin F.
- **C.** Carbaminohaemoglobin.
- **D.** Methaemoglobin.
- **E.** Myohaemoglobin.

1.18 The human fetus can be adversely affected by which of the following maternal situations?
- **A.** Rubella infection.
- **B.** Heparin administered intravenously during the antenatal period.
- **C.** Cigarette smoking.
- **D.** Heroin addiction.
- **E.** Streptomycin therapy during pregnancy.

Answers overleaf

11.15 A, C, D, E.
Vitamin D deficiency is not associated with any type of anaemia. There is no evidence that normal adults require vitamin D in their diet. Rickets may pose obstetrical problems, but anaemia is not one of them.

11.16 A, C, D, E.
Polycythaemia rubra vera is associated with an increased red cell mass, with an expansion in plasma volume if substantial splenomegaly is present. The clinical features are related to increased red cell mass and blood volume changes, not to pulmonary hypertension.

11.17 A, B, C, D.
Myohaemoglobin is a constituent of muscles.

11.18 A, C, D, E.
Heparin has too large a molecule to cross the placenta and therefore there is no affect on the fetus.

.19 The late effects of ionising irradiation to the skin and subcutaneous tissues include:

A. hyperpigmentation.
B. fat atrophy.
C. permanent epilation.
D. depigmentation.
E. infection.

.20 Which of the following characteristically occur in tertiary syphilis?

A. Aortitis.
B. Periostitis.
C. Dissecting aneurysm of the aorta.
D. Lateral column degeneration of the spinal cord.
E. Gummata.

Answers overleaf

11.19 A, B, C, D.
Infection is not a characteristic effect of irradiation to the skin or subcutaneous tissue.

11.20 A, B, E.
Dissecting aneurysms are due to idiopathic cystic medionecrosis and sometimes occur in Marfan's syndrome. Lateral (and posterior) column demyelination is related to vitamin B_{12} deficiency anaemias, not to syphilis. Cerebral syphilis may be meningovascular or parenchymatous. Tabes dorsalis is a degenerative condition of the posterior columns of the spinal cords and posterior roots of the spina[l] nerves.

12. PHARMACOLOGY AND MICROBIOLOGY

.01 The penicillins:
A. interfere with bacterial cell wall synthesis.
B. have a common chemical structure.
C. are excreted in high concentration in urine.
D. when given orally, act more quickly if given after food.
E. are produced by penicillinase.

.02 Ergot alkaloids.
A. Dehydroergotamine causes peripheral venous constriction.
B. Ergotamine antagonises insulin action.
C. They are derivatives of lysergic acid.
D. Ergotism is characterised by peripheral gangrene.
E. They act on the uterus within a minute of an intramuscular injection.

.03 Methyldopa may cause:
A. hypotension.
B. impotence.
C. galactorrhoea.
D. hypokalaemia.
E. bradycardia.

.04 Adrenaline:
A. promotes glycogenolysis in the liver.
B. promotes the entry of triglycerides into adipose tissue.
C. raises diastolic blood pressure.
D. increases heart rate.
E. increases coronary blood flow.

Answers overleaf

12.01 A, C.
The penicillins can be split into five groups: penicillinase-sensitive penicillins, penicillinase-resistant penicillins, broad-spectrum penicillins, antipseudomonal penicillins, and other penicillins. There are also different chemical structures with different substituents into the penicillin and cephalosporin nucleus. Obviously they are not produced by penicillinase. All oral penicillins are best given on an empty stomach to avoid absorption delay caused by food.

12.02 A, C, D.
There is no evidence whatsoever that ergotamine antagonises insulin action. The onset of the effect of ergot alkaloids given intramuscularly is variable, but on average is about 5–10 minutes, with an average of about 7.5 minutes.

12.03 A, B, C, E.
Basic facts. Hypokalaemia does not occur with methyldopa.

12.04 A, D, E.
Adrenaline (and the other catecholamines) promotes the release of fatty acids from triglycerides in adipose tissue, so that the concentration of free fatty acids in the blood increases. The diastolic pressure falls due to the fact that the vascular beds in muscle are dilated.

12.05 Halothane:
A. produces myocardial dysrhythmia.
B. produces liver damage with repetitive anaesthetics.
C. produces bronchial irritation.
D. is a bronchodilator.
E. is non-inflammable.

12.06 Which of the following agents have bronchodilator actions?
A. Pethidine.
B. Morphine.
C. Ether.
D. Salbutamol.
E. Aminophylline.

12.07 Pethidine in therapeutic doses:
A. causes spasm of the biliary sphincter.
B. is metabolised predominently in the liver.
C. is absorbed from the gut.
D. resembles atropine in its action.
E. crosses the placenta.

12.08 The action of coumarin oral anticoagulants may be potentiated by:
A. sulphonamides.
B. salicylates.
C. barbiturates.
D. oral contraceptives.
E. monoamine oxidase inhibitors.

12.09 Suxamethonium (succinylcholine):
A. is rapidly hydrolysed.
B. is a competitive blocker of neuromuscular transmission.
C. has a prolonged action in liver failure.
D. is known to cause muscle pain postoperatively.
E. may cause bradycardia when administered intermittently.

Answers overleaf

12.05 A, B, D, E.
The convenience of halothane as an anaesthetic agent is due to the fact that it is potent and non-irritant. It has three important disadvantages: it causes hypotension, respiratory distress (rapid, shallow breathing), and cardiac arrhythmias (the heart is sensitised to adrenaline and noradrenaline).

12.06 A, C, D, E.
The action of morphine on the bronchial muscle is one of constriction, partly due to histamine release. The effect in general is so slight to be of no importance except in asthmatics.

12.07 A, B, C, D, E.
All basic facts regarding pethidine.

12.08 A, B, E.
Barbiturates and oral contraceptives inhibit the effect of the coumarin oral anticoagulants.

12.09 A, C, D, E.
There are two principal mechanisms by which drugs used clinically interfere with neuromuscular transmission: by competition, and by depolarisation. Suxamethonium is in the latter category.

12.10 Complications of methotrexate therapy are:
- **A.** stomatitis.
- **B.** diarrhoea.
- **C.** tinnitus.
- **D.** alopecia.
- **E.** peripheral neuritis.

12.11 Diseases which may be acquired by skin contact with contaminated water include:
- **A.** schistosomiasis.
- **B.** malaria.
- **C.** leptospirosis (Weil's disease).
- **D.** yellow fever.
- **E.** hydatid disease.

12.12 Fibrinolysins are produced by which of the following organisms?
- **A.** Streptococci.
- **B.** Staphylococci.
- **C.** *Clostridium welchii.*
- **D.** *Mycobacterium tuberculosis.*
- **E.** *Escherichia coli.*

12.13 Vaginal moniliasis:
- **A.** commonly produces pruritus vulvae.
- **B.** is a protozoon infection.
- **C.** can co-exist with *Trichomonas vaginalis*.
- **D.** is eradicated by tetracyclines.
- **E.** is more common in diabetic patients.

Answers overleaf

12.10 A, B, D.
Tinnitus and peripheral neuritis are not recognised complications of methotrexate therapy.

12.11 A, C.
Malaria and yellow fever are transmitted by the mosquito. Hydatid disease is caused by infection resulting from substandard personal hygiene, particularly in sheep farming areas.

12.12 A, B.
Although streptococci and staphylococci produce fibrinolysins, how they contribute to their pathogenicity is not known. Fibrinolysins are not produced by *Mycobacterium tuberculosis*. *Clostridium welchii* produces a powerful exotoxin, and *Esch. coli* produces an endotoxin when dying or dead.

12.13 A, C, E.
Moniliasis is a fungal infection and not erradicated by tetracyclines. The use of oral broad-spectrum antibiotics may be associated with an overgrowth of moniliasis.

12.14 Which of the following organisms may contaminate disinfectants in hospital?

A. *Clostridium welchii.*
B. *Streptococcus viridans.*
C. *Escherichia coli.*
D. *Pseudomonas aeruginosa.*
E. *Staphylococcus pyogenes.*

12.15 Commensal organisms of the vagina include which of the following?

A. Lactobacilli.
B. Streptococci.
C. Yeasts.
D. *Bacteriodes* species.
E. Mycoplasmas.

12.16 *Neisseria gonorrhoeae*:

A. is a diplococcus.
B. may be a commensal in the urethra.
C. may exist in an anaerobic form.
D. requires a moist environment.
E. can be satisfactorily cultured on blood agar.

12.17 Which of the following are Gram-negative?

A. *Clostridium welchii.*
B. *Bacillus proteus.*
C. *Eschericia coli.*
D. *Pseudomonas pyocyanea.*
E. *Streptococcus faecalis.*

Answers overleaf

12.14 A, D.
Staphylococci and streptococci do not contaminate the usual hospital disinfectants and nor does *Esch. coli*.

12.15 A, B, C, D, E.
Almost all known organisms have been found in the vagina as commensals, but only cause problems if they, for one reason or another, reach other parts of the genital tract.

12.16 A, D, E.
The organism is never a commensal, although it may be symptomless. It does not exist in an anaerobic form.

12.17 B, C, D.
Basic facts, certain organisms being Gram-positive or Gram-negative.

12.18 Which of the following conditions may follow streptococcal infection?

A. Acute glomerulonephritis.
B. Rheumatic fever.
C. Lobar pneumonia.
D. Acute osteomyelitis.
E. Acute tonsillitis.

12.19 Which of the following are strict anaerobic organisms?

A. *Clostridium welchii (perfringens).*
B. *Escherichia coli.*
C. *Pseudomonas aeruginosa.*
D. *Actinomyces israeli.*
E. *Clostridium tetani.*

12.20 The effects of viruses include:

A. the production of antibodies.
B. teratogenic effects.
C. the production of interferon.
D. the presence of inclusion bodies in cells.
E. the production of multinucleated giant cells.

Answers overleaf

12.18 A, B, E.
The classic conditions are given. Acute osteomyelitis more commonly follows a staphylococcal infection.

12.19 A, D, E.
Again basic facts regarding strict or obligatory anaerobes.

12.20 A, B, C, D, E.
All acknowledged effects of viruses.

ANSWER SHEETS

	A	B	C	D	E
1	T ⊂⊃ F ⊂⊃	T ⊂⊃ F ⊂⊃	T ⊂⊃ F ⊂⊃	T ⊂⊃ F ⊂⊃	T ⊂⊃ F ⊂⊃
2	T ⊂⊃ F ⊂⊃	T ⊂⊃ F ⊂⊃	T ⊂⊃ F ⊂⊃	T ⊂⊃ F ⊂⊃	T ⊂⊃ F ⊂⊃
3	T ⊂⊃ F ⊂⊃	T ⊂⊃ F ⊂⊃	T ⊂⊃ F ⊂⊃	T ⊂⊃ F ⊂⊃	T ⊂⊃ F ⊂⊃
4	T ⊂⊃ F ⊂⊃	T ⊂⊃ F ⊂⊃	T ⊂⊃ F ⊂⊃	T ⊂⊃ F ⊂⊃	T ⊂⊃ F ⊂⊃
5	T ⊂⊃ F ⊂⊃	T ⊂⊃ F ⊂⊃	T ⊂⊃ F ⊂⊃	T ⊂⊃ F ⊂⊃	T ⊂⊃ F ⊂⊃
6	T ⊂⊃ F ⊂⊃	T ⊂⊃ F ⊂⊃	T ⊂⊃ F ⊂⊃	T ⊂⊃ F ⊂⊃	T ⊂⊃ F ⊂⊃
7	T ⊂⊃ F ⊂⊃	T ⊂⊃ F ⊂⊃	T ⊂⊃ F ⊂⊃	T ⊂⊃ F ⊂⊃	T ⊂⊃ F ⊂⊃
8	T ⊂⊃ F ⊂⊃	T ⊂⊃ F ⊂⊃	T ⊂⊃ F ⊂⊃	T ⊂⊃ F ⊂⊃	T ⊂⊃ F ⊂⊃
9	T ⊂⊃ F ⊂⊃	T ⊂⊃ F ⊂⊃	T ⊂⊃ F ⊂⊃	T ⊂⊃ F ⊂⊃	T ⊂⊃ F ⊂⊃
10	T ⊂⊃ F ⊂⊃	T ⊂⊃ F ⊂⊃	T ⊂⊃ F ⊂⊃	T ⊂⊃ F ⊂⊃	T ⊂⊃ F ⊂⊃

	A	B	C	D	E
11	T ⊂⊃ F ⊂⊃	T ⊂⊃ F ⊂⊃	T ⊂⊃ F ⊂⊃	T ⊂⊃ F ⊂⊃	T ⊂⊃ F ⊂⊃
12	T ⊂⊃ F ⊂⊃	T ⊂⊃ F ⊂⊃	T ⊂⊃ F ⊂⊃	T ⊂⊃ F ⊂⊃	T ⊂⊃ F ⊂⊃
13	T ⊂⊃ F ⊂⊃	T ⊂⊃ F ⊂⊃	T ⊂⊃ F ⊂⊃	T ⊂⊃ F ⊂⊃	T ⊂⊃ F ⊂⊃
14	T ⊂⊃ F ⊂⊃	T ⊂⊃ F ⊂⊃	T ⊂⊃ F ⊂⊃	T ⊂⊃ F ⊂⊃	T ⊂⊃ F ⊂⊃
15	T ⊂⊃ F ⊂⊃	T ⊂⊃ F ⊂⊃	T ⊂⊃ F ⊂⊃	T ⊂⊃ F ⊂⊃	T ⊂⊃ F ⊂⊃
16	T ⊂⊃ F ⊂⊃	T ⊂⊃ F ⊂⊃	T ⊂⊃ F ⊂⊃	T ⊂⊃ F ⊂⊃	T ⊂⊃ F ⊂⊃
17	T ⊂⊃ F ⊂⊃	T ⊂⊃ F ⊂⊃	T ⊂⊃ F ⊂⊃	T ⊂⊃ F ⊂⊃	T ⊂⊃ F ⊂⊃
18	T ⊂⊃ F ⊂⊃	T ⊂⊃ F ⊂⊃	T ⊂⊃ F ⊂⊃	T ⊂⊃ F ⊂⊃	T ⊂⊃ F ⊂⊃
19	T ⊂⊃ F ⊂⊃	T ⊂⊃ F ⊂⊃	T ⊂⊃ F ⊂⊃	T ⊂⊃ F ⊂⊃	T ⊂⊃ F ⊂⊃
20	T ⊂⊃ F ⊂⊃	T ⊂⊃ F ⊂⊃	T ⊂⊃ F ⊂⊃	T ⊂⊃ F ⊂⊃	T ⊂⊃ F ⊂⊃

	A	B	C	D	E
1	T ⊂⊃ F ⊂⊃	T ⊂⊃ F ⊂⊃	T ⊂⊃ F ⊂⊃	T ⊂⊃ F ⊂⊃	T ⊂⊃ F ⊂⊃
2	T ⊂⊃ F ⊂⊃	T ⊂⊃ F ⊂⊃	T ⊂⊃ F ⊂⊃	T ⊂⊃ F ⊂⊃	T ⊂⊃ F ⊂⊃
3	T ⊂⊃ F ⊂⊃	T ⊂⊃ F ⊂⊃	T ⊂⊃ F ⊂⊃	T ⊂⊃ F ⊂⊃	T ⊂⊃ F ⊂⊃
4	T ⊂⊃ F ⊂⊃	T ⊂⊃ F ⊂⊃	T ⊂⊃ F ⊂⊃	T ⊂⊃ F ⊂⊃	T ⊂⊃ F ⊂⊃
5	T ⊂⊃ F ⊂⊃	T ⊂⊃ F ⊂⊃	T ⊂⊃ F ⊂⊃	T ⊂⊃ F ⊂⊃	T ⊂⊃ F ⊂⊃
6	T ⊂⊃ F ⊂⊃	T ⊂⊃ F ⊂⊃	T ⊂⊃ F ⊂⊃	T ⊂⊃ F ⊂⊃	T ⊂⊃ F ⊂⊃
7	T ⊂⊃ F ⊂⊃	T ⊂⊃ F ⊂⊃	T ⊂⊃ F ⊂⊃	T ⊂⊃ F ⊂⊃	T ⊂⊃ F ⊂⊃
8	T ⊂⊃ F ⊂⊃	T ⊂⊃ F ⊂⊃	T ⊂⊃ F ⊂⊃	T ⊂⊃ F ⊂⊃	T ⊂⊃ F ⊂⊃
9	T ⊂⊃ F ⊂⊃	T ⊂⊃ F ⊂⊃	T ⊂⊃ F ⊂⊃	T ⊂⊃ F ⊂⊃	T ⊂⊃ F ⊂⊃
10	T ⊂⊃ F ⊂⊃	T ⊂⊃ F ⊂⊃	T ⊂⊃ F ⊂⊃	T ⊂⊃ F ⊂⊃	T ⊂⊃ F ⊂⊃

	A	B	C	D	E
11	T F	T F	T F	T F	T F
12	T F	T F	T F	T F	T F
13	T F	T F	T F	T F	T F
14	T F	T F	T F	T F	T F
15	T F	T F	T F	T F	T F
16	T F	T F	T F	T F	T F
17	T F	T F	T F	T F	T F
18	T F	T F	T F	T F	T F
19	T F	T F	T F	T F	T F
20	T F	T F	T F	T F	T F

	A	B	C	D	E
1	T ⊂⊃ F ⊂⊃	T ⊂⊃ F ⊂⊃	T ⊂⊃ F ⊂⊃	T ⊂⊃ F ⊂⊃	T ⊂⊃ F ⊂⊃
2	T ⊂⊃ F ⊂⊃	T ⊂⊃ F ⊂⊃	T ⊂⊃ F ⊂⊃	T ⊂⊃ F ⊂⊃	T ⊂⊃ F ⊂⊃
3	T ⊂⊃ F ⊂⊃	T ⊂⊃ F ⊂⊃	T ⊂⊃ F ⊂⊃	T ⊂⊃ F ⊂⊃	T ⊂⊃ F ⊂⊃
4	T ⊂⊃ F ⊂⊃	T ⊂⊃ F ⊂⊃	T ⊂⊃ F ⊂⊃	T ⊂⊃ F ⊂⊃	T ⊂⊃ F ⊂⊃
5	T ⊂⊃ F ⊂⊃	T ⊂⊃ F ⊂⊃	T ⊂⊃ F ⊂⊃	T ⊂⊃ F ⊂⊃	T ⊂⊃ F ⊂⊃
6	T ⊂⊃ F ⊂⊃	T ⊂⊃ F ⊂⊃	T ⊂⊃ F ⊂⊃	T ⊂⊃ F ⊂⊃	T ⊂⊃ F ⊂⊃
7	T ⊂⊃ F ⊂⊃	T ⊂⊃ F ⊂⊃	T ⊂⊃ F ⊂⊃	T ⊂⊃ F ⊂⊃	T ⊂⊃ F ⊂⊃
8	T ⊂⊃ F ⊂⊃	T ⊂⊃ F ⊂⊃	T ⊂⊃ F ⊂⊃	T ⊂⊃ F ⊂⊃	T ⊂⊃ F ⊂⊃
9	T ⊂⊃ F ⊂⊃	T ⊂⊃ F ⊂⊃	T ⊂⊃ F ⊂⊃	T ⊂⊃ F ⊂⊃	T ⊂⊃ F ⊂⊃
10	T ⊂⊃ F ⊂⊃	T ⊂⊃ F ⊂⊃	T ⊂⊃ F ⊂⊃	T ⊂⊃ F ⊂⊃	T ⊂⊃ F ⊂⊃

	A	B	C	D	E
11	T ⊂⊃ F ⊂⊃	T ⊂⊃ F ⊂⊃	T ⊂⊃ F ⊂⊃	T ⊂⊃ F ⊂⊃	T ⊂⊃ F ⊂⊃
12	T ⊂⊃ F ⊂⊃	T ⊂⊃ F ⊂⊃	T ⊂⊃ F ⊂⊃	T ⊂⊃ F ⊂⊃	T ⊂⊃ F ⊂⊃
13	T ⊂⊃ F ⊂⊃	T ⊂⊃ F ⊂⊃	T ⊂⊃ F ⊂⊃	T ⊂⊃ F ⊂⊃	T ⊂⊃ F ⊂⊃
14	T ⊂⊃ F ⊂⊃	T ⊂⊃ F ⊂⊃	T ⊂⊃ F ⊂⊃	T ⊂⊃ F ⊂⊃	T ⊂⊃ F ⊂⊃
15	T ⊂⊃ F ⊂⊃	T ⊂⊃ F ⊂⊃	T ⊂⊃ F ⊂⊃	T ⊂⊃ F ⊂⊃	T ⊂⊃ F ⊂⊃
16	T ⊂⊃ F ⊂⊃	T ⊂⊃ F ⊂⊃	T ⊂⊃ F ⊂⊃	T ⊂⊃ F ⊂⊃	T ⊂⊃ F ⊂⊃
17	T ⊂⊃ F ⊂⊃	T ⊂⊃ F ⊂⊃	T ⊂⊃ F ⊂⊃	T ⊂⊃ F ⊂⊃	T ⊂⊃ F ⊂⊃
18	T ⊂⊃ F ⊂⊃	T ⊂⊃ F ⊂⊃	T ⊂⊃ F ⊂⊃	T ⊂⊃ F ⊂⊃	T ⊂⊃ F ⊂⊃
19	T ⊂⊃ F ⊂⊃	T ⊂⊃ F ⊂⊃	T ⊂⊃ F ⊂⊃	T ⊂⊃ F ⊂⊃	T ⊂⊃ F ⊂⊃
20	T ⊂⊃ F ⊂⊃	T ⊂⊃ F ⊂⊃	T ⊂⊃ F ⊂⊃	T ⊂⊃ F ⊂⊃	T ⊂⊃ F ⊂⊃

1	A T F	B T F	C T F	D T F	E T F
2	A T F	B T F	C T F	D T F	E T F
3	A T F	B T F	C T F	D T F	E T F
4	A T F	B T F	C T F	D T F	E T F
5	A T F	B T F	C T F	D T F	E T F
6	A T F	B T F	C T F	D T F	E T F
7	A T F	B T F	C T F	D T F	E T F
8	A T F	B T F	C T F	D T F	E T F
9	A T F	B T F	C T F	D T F	E T F
10	A T F	B T F	C T F	D T F	E T F

	A	B	C	D	E
11	T ⊂⊃ F ⊂⊃	T ⊂⊃ F ⊂⊃	T ⊂⊃ F ⊂⊃	T ⊂⊃ F ⊂⊃	T ⊂⊃ F ⊂⊃
12	T ⊂⊃ F ⊂⊃	T ⊂⊃ F ⊂⊃	T ⊂⊃ F ⊂⊃	T ⊂⊃ F ⊂⊃	T ⊂⊃ F ⊂⊃
13	T ⊂⊃ F ⊂⊃	T ⊂⊃ F ⊂⊃	T ⊂⊃ F ⊂⊃	T ⊂⊃ F ⊂⊃	T ⊂⊃ F ⊂⊃
14	T ⊂⊃ F ⊂⊃	T ⊂⊃ F ⊂⊃	T ⊂⊃ F ⊂⊃	T ⊂⊃ F ⊂⊃	T ⊂⊃ F ⊂⊃
15	T ⊂⊃ F ⊂⊃	T ⊂⊃ F ⊂⊃	T ⊂⊃ F ⊂⊃	T ⊂⊃ F ⊂⊃	T ⊂⊃ F ⊂⊃
16	T ⊂⊃ F ⊂⊃	T ⊂⊃ F ⊂⊃	T ⊂⊃ F ⊂⊃	T ⊂⊃ F ⊂⊃	T ⊂⊃ F ⊂⊃
17	T ⊂⊃ F ⊂⊃	T ⊂⊃ F ⊂⊃	T ⊂⊃ F ⊂⊃	T ⊂⊃ F ⊂⊃	T ⊂⊃ F ⊂⊃
18	T ⊂⊃ F ⊂⊃	T ⊂⊃ F ⊂⊃	T ⊂⊃ F ⊂⊃	T ⊂⊃ F ⊂⊃	T ⊂⊃ F ⊂⊃
19	T ⊂⊃ F ⊂⊃	T ⊂⊃ F ⊂⊃	T ⊂⊃ F ⊂⊃	T ⊂⊃ F ⊂⊃	T ⊂⊃ F ⊂⊃
20	T ⊂⊃ F ⊂⊃	T ⊂⊃ F ⊂⊃	T ⊂⊃ F ⊂⊃	T ⊂⊃ F ⊂⊃	T ⊂⊃ F ⊂⊃

	A	B	C	D	E
1	T ⊂⊃ F ⊂⊃	T ⊂⊃ F ⊂⊃	T ⊂⊃ F ⊂⊃	T ⊂⊃ F ⊂⊃	T ⊂⊃ F ⊂⊃
2	T ⊂⊃ F ⊂⊃	T ⊂⊃ F ⊂⊃	T ⊂⊃ F ⊂⊃	T ⊂⊃ F ⊂⊃	T ⊂⊃ F ⊂⊃
3	T ⊂⊃ F ⊂⊃	T ⊂⊃ F ⊂⊃	T ⊂⊃ F ⊂⊃	T ⊂⊃ F ⊂⊃	T ⊂⊃ F ⊂⊃
4	T ⊂⊃ F ⊂⊃	T ⊂⊃ F ⊂⊃	T ⊂⊃ F ⊂⊃	T ⊂⊃ F ⊂⊃	T ⊂⊃ F ⊂⊃
5	T ⊂⊃ F ⊂⊃	T ⊂⊃ F ⊂⊃	T ⊂⊃ F ⊂⊃	T ⊂⊃ F ⊂⊃	T ⊂⊃ F ⊂⊃
6	T ⊂⊃ F ⊂⊃	T ⊂⊃ F ⊂⊃	T ⊂⊃ F ⊂⊃	T ⊂⊃ F ⊂⊃	T ⊂⊃ F ⊂⊃
7	T ⊂⊃ F ⊂⊃	T ⊂⊃ F ⊂⊃	T ⊂⊃ F ⊂⊃	T ⊂⊃ F ⊂⊃	T ⊂⊃ F ⊂⊃
8	T ⊂⊃ F ⊂⊃	T ⊂⊃ F ⊂⊃	T ⊂⊃ F ⊂⊃	T ⊂⊃ F ⊂⊃	T ⊂⊃ F ⊂⊃
9	T ⊂⊃ F ⊂⊃	T ⊂⊃ F ⊂⊃	T ⊂⊃ F ⊂⊃	T ⊂⊃ F ⊂⊃	T ⊂⊃ F ⊂⊃
10	T ⊂⊃ F ⊂⊃	T ⊂⊃ F ⊂⊃	T ⊂⊃ F ⊂⊃	T ⊂⊃ F ⊂⊃	T ⊂⊃ F ⊂⊃

	A	B	C	D	E
11	T ⊂⊃ F ⊂⊃	T ⊂⊃ F ⊂⊃	T ⊂⊃ F ⊂⊃	T ⊂⊃ F ⊂⊃	T ⊂⊃ F ⊂⊃
12	T ⊂⊃ F ⊂⊃	T ⊂⊃ F ⊂⊃	T ⊂⊃ F ⊂⊃	T ⊂⊃ F ⊂⊃	T ⊂⊃ F ⊂⊃
13	T ⊂⊃ F ⊂⊃	T ⊂⊃ F ⊂⊃	T ⊂⊃ F ⊂⊃	T ⊂⊃ F ⊂⊃	T ⊂⊃ F ⊂⊃
14	T ⊂⊃ F ⊂⊃	T ⊂⊃ F ⊂⊃	T ⊂⊃ F ⊂⊃	T ⊂⊃ F ⊂⊃	T ⊂⊃ F ⊂⊃
15	T ⊂⊃ F ⊂⊃	T ⊂⊃ F ⊂⊃	T ⊂⊃ F ⊂⊃	T ⊂⊃ F ⊂⊃	T ⊂⊃ F ⊂⊃
16	T ⊂⊃ F ⊂⊃	T ⊂⊃ F ⊂⊃	T ⊂⊃ F ⊂⊃	T ⊂⊃ F ⊂⊃	T ⊂⊃ F ⊂⊃
17	T ⊂⊃ F ⊂⊃	T ⊂⊃ F ⊂⊃	T ⊂⊃ F ⊂⊃	T ⊂⊃ F ⊂⊃	T ⊂⊃ F ⊂⊃
18	T ⊂⊃ F ⊂⊃	T ⊂⊃ F ⊂⊃	T ⊂⊃ F ⊂⊃	T ⊂⊃ F ⊂⊃	T ⊂⊃ F ⊂⊃
19	T ⊂⊃ F ⊂⊃	T ⊂⊃ F ⊂⊃	T ⊂⊃ F ⊂⊃	T ⊂⊃ F ⊂⊃	T ⊂⊃ F ⊂⊃
20	T ⊂⊃ F ⊂⊃	T ⊂⊃ F ⊂⊃	T ⊂⊃ F ⊂⊃	T ⊂⊃ F ⊂⊃	T ⊂⊃ F ⊂⊃

	A	B	C	D	E
1	T ⊂⊃ F ⊂⊃	T ⊂⊃ F ⊂⊃	T ⊂⊃ F ⊂⊃	T ⊂⊃ F ⊂⊃	T ⊂⊃ F ⊂⊃
2	T ⊂⊃ F ⊂⊃	T ⊂⊃ F ⊂⊃	T ⊂⊃ F ⊂⊃	T ⊂⊃ F ⊂⊃	T ⊂⊃ F ⊂⊃
3	T ⊂⊃ F ⊂⊃	T ⊂⊃ F ⊂⊃	T ⊂⊃ F ⊂⊃	T ⊂⊃ F ⊂⊃	T ⊂⊃ F ⊂⊃
4	T ⊂⊃ F ⊂⊃	T ⊂⊃ F ⊂⊃	T ⊂⊃ F ⊂⊃	T ⊂⊃ F ⊂⊃	T ⊂⊃ F ⊂⊃
5	T ⊂⊃ F ⊂⊃	T ⊂⊃ F ⊂⊃	T ⊂⊃ F ⊂⊃	T ⊂⊃ F ⊂⊃	T ⊂⊃ F ⊂⊃
6	T ⊂⊃ F ⊂⊃	T ⊂⊃ F ⊂⊃	T ⊂⊃ F ⊂⊃	T ⊂⊃ F ⊂⊃	T ⊂⊃ F ⊂⊃
7	T ⊂⊃ F ⊂⊃	T ⊂⊃ F ⊂⊃	T ⊂⊃ F ⊂⊃	T ⊂⊃ F ⊂⊃	T ⊂⊃ F ⊂⊃
8	T ⊂⊃ F ⊂⊃	T ⊂⊃ F ⊂⊃	T ⊂⊃ F ⊂⊃	T ⊂⊃ F ⊂⊃	T ⊂⊃ F ⊂⊃
9	T ⊂⊃ F ⊂⊃	T ⊂⊃ F ⊂⊃	T ⊂⊃ F ⊂⊃	T ⊂⊃ F ⊂⊃	T ⊂⊃ F ⊂⊃
10	T ⊂⊃ F ⊂⊃	T ⊂⊃ F ⊂⊃	T ⊂⊃ F ⊂⊃	T ⊂⊃ F ⊂⊃	T ⊂⊃ F ⊂⊃

	A	B	C	D	E
11	T ⊂⊃ F ⊂⊃	T ⊂⊃ F ⊂⊃	T ⊂⊃ F ⊂⊃	T ⊂⊃ F ⊂⊃	T ⊂⊃ F ⊂⊃
12	T ⊂⊃ F ⊂⊃	T ⊂⊃ F ⊂⊃	T ⊂⊃ F ⊂⊃	T ⊂⊃ F ⊂⊃	T ⊂⊃ F ⊂⊃
13	T ⊂⊃ F ⊂⊃	T ⊂⊃ F ⊂⊃	T ⊂⊃ F ⊂⊃	T ⊂⊃ F ⊂⊃	T ⊂⊃ F ⊂⊃
14	T ⊂⊃ F ⊂⊃	T ⊂⊃ F ⊂⊃	T ⊂⊃ F ⊂⊃	T ⊂⊃ F ⊂⊃	T ⊂⊃ F ⊂⊃
15	T ⊂⊃ F ⊂⊃	T ⊂⊃ F ⊂⊃	T ⊂⊃ F ⊂⊃	T ⊂⊃ F ⊂⊃	T ⊂⊃ F ⊂⊃
16	T ⊂⊃ F ⊂⊃	T ⊂⊃ F ⊂⊃	T ⊂⊃ F ⊂⊃	T ⊂⊃ F ⊂⊃	T ⊂⊃ F ⊂⊃
17	T ⊂⊃ F ⊂⊃	T ⊂⊃ F ⊂⊃	T ⊂⊃ F ⊂⊃	T ⊂⊃ F ⊂⊃	T ⊂⊃ F ⊂⊃
18	T ⊂⊃ F ⊂⊃	T ⊂⊃ F ⊂⊃	T ⊂⊃ F ⊂⊃	T ⊂⊃ F ⊂⊃	T ⊂⊃ F ⊂⊃
19	T ⊂⊃ F ⊂⊃	T ⊂⊃ F ⊂⊃	T ⊂⊃ F ⊂⊃	T ⊂⊃ F ⊂⊃	T ⊂⊃ F ⊂⊃
20	T ⊂⊃ F ⊂⊃	T ⊂⊃ F ⊂⊃	T ⊂⊃ F ⊂⊃	T ⊂⊃ F ⊂⊃	T ⊂⊃ F ⊂⊃

	A	B	C	D	E
1	T ⊂⊃ F ⊂⊃	T ⊂⊃ F ⊂⊃	T ⊂⊃ F ⊂⊃	T ⊂⊃ F ⊂⊃	T ⊂⊃ F ⊂⊃
2	T ⊂⊃ F ⊂⊃	T ⊂⊃ F ⊂⊃	T ⊂⊃ F ⊂⊃	T ⊂⊃ F ⊂⊃	T ⊂⊃ F ⊂⊃
3	T ⊂⊃ F ⊂⊃	T ⊂⊃ F ⊂⊃	T ⊂⊃ F ⊂⊃	T ⊂⊃ F ⊂⊃	T ⊂⊃ F ⊂⊃
4	T ⊂⊃ F ⊂⊃	T ⊂⊃ F ⊂⊃	T ⊂⊃ F ⊂⊃	T ⊂⊃ F ⊂⊃	T ⊂⊃ F ⊂⊃
5	T ⊂⊃ F ⊂⊃	T ⊂⊃ F ⊂⊃	T ⊂⊃ F ⊂⊃	T ⊂⊃ F ⊂⊃	T ⊂⊃ F ⊂⊃
6	T ⊂⊃ F ⊂⊃	T ⊂⊃ F ⊂⊃	T ⊂⊃ F ⊂⊃	T ⊂⊃ F ⊂⊃	T ⊂⊃ F ⊂⊃
7	T ⊂⊃ F ⊂⊃	T ⊂⊃ F ⊂⊃	T ⊂⊃ F ⊂⊃	T ⊂⊃ F ⊂⊃	T ⊂⊃ F ⊂⊃
8	T ⊂⊃ F ⊂⊃	T ⊂⊃ F ⊂⊃	T ⊂⊃ F ⊂⊃	T ⊂⊃ F ⊂⊃	T ⊂⊃ F ⊂⊃
9	T ⊂⊃ F ⊂⊃	T ⊂⊃ F ⊂⊃	T ⊂⊃ F ⊂⊃	T ⊂⊃ F ⊂⊃	T ⊂⊃ F ⊂⊃
10	T ⊂⊃ F ⊂⊃	T ⊂⊃ F ⊂⊃	T ⊂⊃ F ⊂⊃	T ⊂⊃ F ⊂⊃	T ⊂⊃ F ⊂⊃

	A	B	C	D	E
11	T F	T F	T F	T F	T F
12	T F	T F	T F	T F	T F
13	T F	T F	T F	T F	T F
14	T F	T F	T F	T F	T F
15	T F	T F	T F	T F	T F
16	T F	T F	T F	T F	T F
17	T F	T F	T F	T F	T F
18	T F	T F	T F	T F	T F
19	T F	T F	T F	T F	T F
20	T F	T F	T F	T F	T F

1	A T F	B T F	C T F	D T F	E T F
2	A T F	B T F	C T F	D T F	E T F
3	A T F	B T F	C T F	D T F	E T F
4	A T F	B T F	C T F	D T F	E T F
5	A T F	B T F	C T F	D T F	E T F
6	A T F	B T F	C T F	D T F	E T F
7	A T F	B T F	C T F	D T F	E T F
8	A T F	B T F	C T F	D T F	E T F
9	A T F	B T F	C T F	D T F	E T F
10	A T F	B T F	C T F	D T F	E T F

	A	B	C	D	E
11	T ⊂⊃ F ⊂⊃	T ⊂⊃ F ⊂⊃	T ⊂⊃ F ⊂⊃	T ⊂⊃ F ⊂⊃	T ⊂⊃ F ⊂⊃
12	T ⊂⊃ F ⊂⊃	T ⊂⊃ F ⊂⊃	T ⊂⊃ F ⊂⊃	T ⊂⊃ F ⊂⊃	T ⊂⊃ F ⊂⊃
13	T ⊂⊃ F ⊂⊃	T ⊂⊃ F ⊂⊃	T ⊂⊃ F ⊂⊃	T ⊂⊃ F ⊂⊃	T ⊂⊃ F ⊂⊃
14	T ⊂⊃ F ⊂⊃	T ⊂⊃ F ⊂⊃	T ⊂⊃ F ⊂⊃	T ⊂⊃ F ⊂⊃	T ⊂⊃ F ⊂⊃
15	T ⊂⊃ F ⊂⊃	T ⊂⊃ F ⊂⊃	T ⊂⊃ F ⊂⊃	T ⊂⊃ F ⊂⊃	T ⊂⊃ F ⊂⊃
16	T ⊂⊃ F ⊂⊃	T ⊂⊃ F ⊂⊃	T ⊂⊃ F ⊂⊃	T ⊂⊃ F ⊂⊃	T ⊂⊃ F ⊂⊃
17	T ⊂⊃ F ⊂⊃	T ⊂⊃ F ⊂⊃	T ⊂⊃ F ⊂⊃	T ⊂⊃ F ⊂⊃	T ⊂⊃ F ⊂⊃
18	T ⊂⊃ F ⊂⊃	T ⊂⊃ F ⊂⊃	T ⊂⊃ F ⊂⊃	T ⊂⊃ F ⊂⊃	T ⊂⊃ F ⊂⊃
19	T ⊂⊃ F ⊂⊃	T ⊂⊃ F ⊂⊃	T ⊂⊃ F ⊂⊃	T ⊂⊃ F ⊂⊃	T ⊂⊃ F ⊂⊃
20	T ⊂⊃ F ⊂⊃	T ⊂⊃ F ⊂⊃	T ⊂⊃ F ⊂⊃	T ⊂⊃ F ⊂⊃	T ⊂⊃ F ⊂⊃

	A	B	C	D	E
1	T F	T F	T F	T F	T F
2	T F	T F	T F	T F	T F
3	T F	T F	T F	T F	T F
4	T F	T F	T F	T F	T F
5	T F	T F	T F	T F	T F
6	T F	T F	T F	T F	T F
7	T F	T F	T F	T F	T F
8	T F	T F	T F	T F	T F
9	T F	T F	T F	T F	T F
10	T F	T F	T F	T F	T F

	A	B	C	D	E
11	T ⊂⊃ F ⊂⊃	T ⊂⊃ F ⊂⊃	T ⊂⊃ F ⊂⊃	T ⊂⊃ F ⊂⊃	T ⊂⊃ F ⊂⊃
12	T ⊂⊃ F ⊂⊃	T ⊂⊃ F ⊂⊃	T ⊂⊃ F ⊂⊃	T ⊂⊃ F ⊂⊃	T ⊂⊃ F ⊂⊃
13	T ⊂⊃ F ⊂⊃	T ⊂⊃ F ⊂⊃	T ⊂⊃ F ⊂⊃	T ⊂⊃ F ⊂⊃	T ⊂⊃ F ⊂⊃
14	T ⊂⊃ F ⊂⊃	T ⊂⊃ F ⊂⊃	T ⊂⊃ F ⊂⊃	T ⊂⊃ F ⊂⊃	T ⊂⊃ F ⊂⊃
15	T ⊂⊃ F ⊂⊃	T ⊂⊃ F ⊂⊃	T ⊂⊃ F ⊂⊃	T ⊂⊃ F ⊂⊃	T ⊂⊃ F ⊂⊃
16	T ⊂⊃ F ⊂⊃	T ⊂⊃ F ⊂⊃	T ⊂⊃ F ⊂⊃	T ⊂⊃ F ⊂⊃	T ⊂⊃ F ⊂⊃
17	T ⊂⊃ F ⊂⊃	T ⊂⊃ F ⊂⊃	T ⊂⊃ F ⊂⊃	T ⊂⊃ F ⊂⊃	T ⊂⊃ F ⊂⊃
18	T ⊂⊃ F ⊂⊃	T ⊂⊃ F ⊂⊃	T ⊂⊃ F ⊂⊃	T ⊂⊃ F ⊂⊃	T ⊂⊃ F ⊂⊃
19	T ⊂⊃ F ⊂⊃	T ⊂⊃ F ⊂⊃	T ⊂⊃ F ⊂⊃	T ⊂⊃ F ⊂⊃	T ⊂⊃ F ⊂⊃
20	T ⊂⊃ F ⊂⊃	T ⊂⊃ F ⊂⊃	T ⊂⊃ F ⊂⊃	T ⊂⊃ F ⊂⊃	T ⊂⊃ F ⊂⊃

1	A T F	B T F	C T F	D T F	E T F
2	A T F	B T F	C T F	D T F	E T F
3	A T F	B T F	C T F	D T F	E T F
4	A T F	B T F	C T F	D T F	E T F
5	A T F	B T F	C T F	D T F	E T F
6	A T F	B T F	C T F	D T F	E T F
7	A T F	B T F	C T F	D T F	E T F
8	A T F	B T F	C T F	D T F	E T F
9	A T F	B T F	C T F	D T F	E T F
10	A T F	B T F	C T F	D T F	E T F

	A	B	C	D	E
11	T ⊂⊃ F ⊂⊃	T ⊂⊃ F ⊂⊃	T ⊂⊃ F ⊂⊃	T ⊂⊃ F ⊂⊃	T ⊂⊃ F ⊂⊃
12	T ⊂⊃ F ⊂⊃	T ⊂⊃ F ⊂⊃	T ⊂⊃ F ⊂⊃	T ⊂⊃ F ⊂⊃	T ⊂⊃ F ⊂⊃
13	T ⊂⊃ F ⊂⊃	T ⊂⊃ F ⊂⊃	T ⊂⊃ F ⊂⊃	T ⊂⊃ F ⊂⊃	T ⊂⊃ F ⊂⊃
14	T ⊂⊃ F ⊂⊃	T ⊂⊃ F ⊂⊃	T ⊂⊃ F ⊂⊃	T ⊂⊃ F ⊂⊃	T ⊂⊃ F ⊂⊃
15	T ⊂⊃ F ⊂⊃	T ⊂⊃ F ⊂⊃	T ⊂⊃ F ⊂⊃	T ⊂⊃ F ⊂⊃	T ⊂⊃ F ⊂⊃
16	T ⊂⊃ F ⊂⊃	T ⊂⊃ F ⊂⊃	T ⊂⊃ F ⊂⊃	T ⊂⊃ F ⊂⊃	T ⊂⊃ F ⊂⊃
17	T ⊂⊃ F ⊂⊃	T ⊂⊃ F ⊂⊃	T ⊂⊃ F ⊂⊃	T ⊂⊃ F ⊂⊃	T ⊂⊃ F ⊂⊃
18	T ⊂⊃ F ⊂⊃	T ⊂⊃ F ⊂⊃	T ⊂⊃ F ⊂⊃	T ⊂⊃ F ⊂⊃	T ⊂⊃ F ⊂⊃
19	T ⊂⊃ F ⊂⊃	T ⊂⊃ F ⊂⊃	T ⊂⊃ F ⊂⊃	T ⊂⊃ F ⊂⊃	T ⊂⊃ F ⊂⊃
20	T ⊂⊃ F ⊂⊃	T ⊂⊃ F ⊂⊃	T ⊂⊃ F ⊂⊃	T ⊂⊃ F ⊂⊃	T ⊂⊃ F ⊂⊃

	A	B	C	D	E
1	T ⊂⊃ F ⊂⊃	T ⊂⊃ F ⊂⊃	T ⊂⊃ F ⊂⊃	T ⊂⊃ F ⊂⊃	T ⊂⊃ F ⊂⊃
2	T ⊂⊃ F ⊂⊃	T ⊂⊃ F ⊂⊃	T ⊂⊃ F ⊂⊃	T ⊂⊃ F ⊂⊃	T ⊂⊃ F ⊂⊃
3	T ⊂⊃ F ⊂⊃	T ⊂⊃ F ⊂⊃	T ⊂⊃ F ⊂⊃	T ⊂⊃ F ⊂⊃	T ⊂⊃ F ⊂⊃
4	T ⊂⊃ F ⊂⊃	T ⊂⊃ F ⊂⊃	T ⊂⊃ F ⊂⊃	T ⊂⊃ F ⊂⊃	T ⊂⊃ F ⊂⊃
5	T ⊂⊃ F ⊂⊃	T ⊂⊃ F ⊂⊃	T ⊂⊃ F ⊂⊃	T ⊂⊃ F ⊂⊃	T ⊂⊃ F ⊂⊃
6	T ⊂⊃ F ⊂⊃	T ⊂⊃ F ⊂⊃	T ⊂⊃ F ⊂⊃	T ⊂⊃ F ⊂⊃	T ⊂⊃ F ⊂⊃
7	T ⊂⊃ F ⊂⊃	T ⊂⊃ F ⊂⊃	T ⊂⊃ F ⊂⊃	T ⊂⊃ F ⊂⊃	T ⊂⊃ F ⊂⊃
8	T ⊂⊃ F ⊂⊃	T ⊂⊃ F ⊂⊃	T ⊂⊃ F ⊂⊃	T ⊂⊃ F ⊂⊃	T ⊂⊃ F ⊂⊃
9	T ⊂⊃ F ⊂⊃	T ⊂⊃ F ⊂⊃	T ⊂⊃ F ⊂⊃	T ⊂⊃ F ⊂⊃	T ⊂⊃ F ⊂⊃
10	T ⊂⊃ F ⊂⊃	T ⊂⊃ F ⊂⊃	T ⊂⊃ F ⊂⊃	T ⊂⊃ F ⊂⊃	T ⊂⊃ F ⊂⊃

	A	B	C	D	E
11	T ⊂⊃ F ⊂⊃	T ⊂⊃ F ⊂⊃	T ⊂⊃ F ⊂⊃	T ⊂⊃ F ⊂⊃	T ⊂⊃ F ⊂⊃
12	T ⊂⊃ F ⊂⊃	T ⊂⊃ F ⊂⊃	T ⊂⊃ F ⊂⊃	T ⊂⊃ F ⊂⊃	T ⊂⊃ F ⊂⊃
13	T ⊂⊃ F ⊂⊃	T ⊂⊃ F ⊂⊃	T ⊂⊃ F ⊂⊃	T ⊂⊃ F ⊂⊃	T ⊂⊃ F ⊂⊃
14	T ⊂⊃ F ⊂⊃	T ⊂⊃ F ⊂⊃	T ⊂⊃ F ⊂⊃	T ⊂⊃ F ⊂⊃	T ⊂⊃ F ⊂⊃
15	T ⊂⊃ F ⊂⊃	T ⊂⊃ F ⊂⊃	T ⊂⊃ F ⊂⊃	T ⊂⊃ F ⊂⊃	T ⊂⊃ F ⊂⊃
16	T ⊂⊃ F ⊂⊃	T ⊂⊃ F ⊂⊃	T ⊂⊃ F ⊂⊃	T ⊂⊃ F ⊂⊃	T ⊂⊃ F ⊂⊃
17	T ⊂⊃ F ⊂⊃	T ⊂⊃ F ⊂⊃	T ⊂⊃ F ⊂⊃	T ⊂⊃ F ⊂⊃	T ⊂⊃ F ⊂⊃
18	T ⊂⊃ F ⊂⊃	T ⊂⊃ F ⊂⊃	T ⊂⊃ F ⊂⊃	T ⊂⊃ F ⊂⊃	T ⊂⊃ F ⊂⊃
19	T ⊂⊃ F ⊂⊃	T ⊂⊃ F ⊂⊃	T ⊂⊃ F ⊂⊃	T ⊂⊃ F ⊂⊃	T ⊂⊃ F ⊂⊃
20	T ⊂⊃ F ⊂⊃	T ⊂⊃ F ⊂⊃	T ⊂⊃ F ⊂⊃	T ⊂⊃ F ⊂⊃	T ⊂⊃ F ⊂⊃

	A	B	C	D	E
1	T ⊂⊃ F ⊂⊃	T ⊂⊃ F ⊂⊃	T ⊂⊃ F ⊂⊃	T ⊂⊃ F ⊂⊃	T ⊂⊃ F ⊂⊃
2	T ⊂⊃ F ⊂⊃	T ⊂⊃ F ⊂⊃	T ⊂⊃ F ⊂⊃	T ⊂⊃ F ⊂⊃	T ⊂⊃ F ⊂⊃
3	T ⊂⊃ F ⊂⊃	T ⊂⊃ F ⊂⊃	T ⊂⊃ F ⊂⊃	T ⊂⊃ F ⊂⊃	T ⊂⊃ F ⊂⊃
4	T ⊂⊃ F ⊂⊃	T ⊂⊃ F ⊂⊃	T ⊂⊃ F ⊂⊃	T ⊂⊃ F ⊂⊃	T ⊂⊃ F ⊂⊃
5	T ⊂⊃ F ⊂⊃	T ⊂⊃ F ⊂⊃	T ⊂⊃ F ⊂⊃	T ⊂⊃ F ⊂⊃	T ⊂⊃ F ⊂⊃
6	T ⊂⊃ F ⊂⊃	T ⊂⊃ F ⊂⊃	T ⊂⊃ F ⊂⊃	T ⊂⊃ F ⊂⊃	T ⊂⊃ F ⊂⊃
7	T ⊂⊃ F ⊂⊃	T ⊂⊃ F ⊂⊃	T ⊂⊃ F ⊂⊃	T ⊂⊃ F ⊂⊃	T ⊂⊃ F ⊂⊃
8	T ⊂⊃ F ⊂⊃	T ⊂⊃ F ⊂⊃	T ⊂⊃ F ⊂⊃	T ⊂⊃ F ⊂⊃	T ⊂⊃ F ⊂⊃
9	T ⊂⊃ F ⊂⊃	T ⊂⊃ F ⊂⊃	T ⊂⊃ F ⊂⊃	T ⊂⊃ F ⊂⊃	T ⊂⊃ F ⊂⊃
10	T ⊂⊃ F ⊂⊃	T ⊂⊃ F ⊂⊃	T ⊂⊃ F ⊂⊃	T ⊂⊃ F ⊂⊃	T ⊂⊃ F ⊂⊃

	A	B	C	D	E
11	T ⊂⊃ F ⊂⊃	T ⊂⊃ F ⊂⊃	T ⊂⊃ F ⊂⊃	T ⊂⊃ F ⊂⊃	T ⊂⊃ F ⊂⊃
12	T ⊂⊃ F ⊂⊃	T ⊂⊃ F ⊂⊃	T ⊂⊃ F ⊂⊃	T ⊂⊃ F ⊂⊃	T ⊂⊃ F ⊂⊃
13	T ⊂⊃ F ⊂⊃	T ⊂⊃ F ⊂⊃	T ⊂⊃ F ⊂⊃	T ⊂⊃ F ⊂⊃	T ⊂⊃ F ⊂⊃
14	T ⊂⊃ F ⊂⊃	T ⊂⊃ F ⊂⊃	T ⊂⊃ F ⊂⊃	T ⊂⊃ F ⊂⊃	T ⊂⊃ F ⊂⊃
15	T ⊂⊃ F ⊂⊃	T ⊂⊃ F ⊂⊃	T ⊂⊃ F ⊂⊃	T ⊂⊃ F ⊂⊃	T ⊂⊃ F ⊂⊃
16	T ⊂⊃ F ⊂⊃	T ⊂⊃ F ⊂⊃	T ⊂⊃ F ⊂⊃	T ⊂⊃ F ⊂⊃	T ⊂⊃ F ⊂⊃
17	T ⊂⊃ F ⊂⊃	T ⊂⊃ F ⊂⊃	T ⊂⊃ F ⊂⊃	T ⊂⊃ F ⊂⊃	T ⊂⊃ F ⊂⊃
18	T ⊂⊃ F ⊂⊃	T ⊂⊃ F ⊂⊃	T ⊂⊃ F ⊂⊃	T ⊂⊃ F ⊂⊃	T ⊂⊃ F ⊂⊃
19	T ⊂⊃ F ⊂⊃	T ⊂⊃ F ⊂⊃	T ⊂⊃ F ⊂⊃	T ⊂⊃ F ⊂⊃	T ⊂⊃ F ⊂⊃
20	T ⊂⊃ F ⊂⊃	T ⊂⊃ F ⊂⊃	T ⊂⊃ F ⊂⊃	T ⊂⊃ F ⊂⊃	T ⊂⊃ F ⊂⊃